Lecture Notes in Computer Science 10081

Commenced Publication in 1973
Founding and Former Series Editors:
Gerhard Goos, Juris Hartmanis, and Jan van Leeuwen

Henning Müller · B. Michael Kelm
Tal Arbel · Weidong Cai
M. Jorge Cardoso · Georg Langs
Bjoern Menze · Dimitris Metaxas
Albert Montillo · William M. Wells III
Shaoting Zhang · Albert C.S. Chung
Mark Jenkinson · Annemie Ribbens (Eds.)

Medical Computer Vision and Bayesian and Graphical Models for Biomedical Imaging

MICCAI 2016 International Workshops, MCV and BAMBI
Athens, Greece, October 21, 2016
Revised Selected Papers

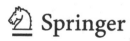 Springer

Editors

Henning Müller
HES-SO
Sierre, Switzerland

B. Michael Kelm
Siemens AG
Munich, Germany

Tal Arbel
McGill University
Montreal, QC, Canada

Weidong Cai
University of Sydney
Sydney, NSW, Australia

M. Jorge Cardoso
University College London
London, UK

Georg Langs
Medical University of Vienna
Vienna, Austria

Bjoern Menze
Technische Universität München
Garching, Germany

Dimitris Metaxas
Rutgers The State University of New Jersey
Piscataway, NJ, USA

Albert Montillo
University of Texas Southwestern Medical Center
Dallas, TX, USA

William M. Wells III
Brigham and Women's Hospital
Boston, MA, USA

Shaoting Zhang
University of North Carolina at Charlotte
Charlotte, NC, USA

Albert C.S. Chung
The Hong Kong University of Science
    and Technology
Clear Water Bay, Hong Kong, SAR China

Mark Jenkinson
University of Oxford
John Radcliffe Hospital
Oxford, UK

Annemie Ribbens
IcoMetrix
Leuven, Belgium

ISSN 0302-9743   ISSN 1611-3349   (electronic)
Lecture Notes in Computer Science
ISBN 978-3-319-61187-7   ISBN 978-3-319-61188-4   (eBook)
DOI 10.1007/978-3-319-61188-4

Library of Congress Control Number: 2017943850

LNCS Sublibrary: SL6 – Image Processing, Computer Vision, Pattern Recognition, and Graphics

Printed on acid-free paper

This Springer imprint is published by Springer Nature
The registered company is Springer International Publishing AG
The registered company address is: Gewerbestrasse 11, 6330 Cham, Switzerland

Preface MCV 2016

The MICCAI 2016 Workshop on Medical Computer Vision: Algorithms for Big Data (MCV 2016) was held in conjunction with the 19th International Conference on Medical Image Computing and Computer-Assisted Intervention (MICCAI 2016) on October 21, 2016, in Athens, Greece. It succeeded the workshops on Medical Computer Vision that were held in September 2010 in conjunction with MICCAI 2010 in Beijing, in June 2012 in conjunction with CVPR 2012 in Providence, in October 2012 in conjunction with MICCAI 2012 in Nice, in September 2013 in conjunction with MICCAI 2013 in Nagoya, in September 2014 in conjunction with MICCAI 2014 in Boston, and in June 2015 in conjunction with CVPR 2015 in Boston.

Modern learning algorithms make the promise of bridging the semantic gap between images and diagnoses and even reaching superhuman performance. The goal of this workshop is to explore the use of "big data" algorithms for harvesting, organizing and learning from large-scale medical imaging data sets and for general-purpose automatic understanding of medical images. This includes modern, scalable, and efficient algorithms for automatic localization, segmentation, registration, and characterization of anatomical features and anomalies. We are especially interested in new methodology strongly motivated by a clinical application with a contribution at the interface of big data algorithms, computer vision, machine learning, and medical image analysis.

Our call for papers resulted in 15 submissions of up to 12 pages. Each paper received two to four reviews. Based on these peer reviews, we accepted 13 papers to the workshop among which six were assigned a long and seven a short oral presentation.

Six invited speakers (Wiro Niessen, Kevin Zhou, Geert Litjens, Mert Sabuncu, Sandy Wells, Ben Glocker) also made major contributions to the program. The many questions and discussions showed the quality of the talks and the posters. Particularly the use of large data sets was much discussed, something that is not easy to obtain with annotations in the medical field. The large participation reflected the interest of the public in the workshop topics.

October 2016

Henning Müller
Michael Kelm
Weidong Cai
Georg Langs
Bjoern Menze
Dimitris Metaxas
Albert Montillo
Shaoting Zhang

Preface BAMBI 2016

BAMBI 2016 was the Third International Workshop on Bayesian and Graphical Models for Biomedical Imaging. It was held at the Intercontinental Athenaeum, Arcade I, Athens, Greece, on October 21, 2016. The goal of this event was to highlight the potential of using Bayesian or random field graphical models for advancing scientific research in biomedical image analysis. The BAMBI 2016 proceedings, published in the *Lecture Notes in Computer Science* series together with the Medical Computer Vision workshop, contain state-of-the-art original and highly methodological research selected through a rigorous peer-review process. Every full paper went through a double-blind review process by at least three members of the international Program Committee composed of several renowned scientists in the field of Bayesian image analysis. The result of this stringent selection process was a set of six articles in a single-track single-day event.

The scientific program was augmented by our two invited speakers, Mark Jenkinson (Nuffield Department of Clinical Neurosciences, Oxford University, Oxford, UK) and Ben Glocker (Imperial College London, London, UK). Both presented exciting advances during their keynote lectures, covering a large scope of methodologies and applications in Bayesian and graphical models. We warmly thank the members of our Program Committee and all the participants of the event who made this workshop an exciting venue to share the latest methodological advances in this expanding research area.

October 2016

Tal Arbel
M. Jorge Cardoso
Albert C.S. Chung
Mark Jenkinson
Annemie Ribbens
William M. Wells III

Organization

Organizing Committee MCV 2016

General Co-chairs

Michael Kelm, Germany
Bjoern Menze, Germany
Georg Langs, Austria
Albert Montillo, USA
Henning Müller, Switzerland
Shaoting Zhang, USA
Weidong Cai, Australia
Dimitris Metaxas, USA

Publication Chair

Henning Müller, Switzerland

Organizing Committee BAMBI 2016

Co-chairs

Tal Arbel, Canada
M. Jorge Cardoso, UK
Albert C.S. Chung, Hong Kong, SAR China
Mark Jenkinson, UK
Annemie Ribbens, Belgium
William M. Wells III, USA

International Program Committee MCV 2016

Adrien Depeursinge	HES-SO and EPFL, Switzerland
Alison Nobel	University of Oxford, UK
Cagatay Demiralp	Stanford University, USA
Christian Barrillot	IRISA Rennes, France
Diana Mateus	TU Munich, Germany
Dinggang Shen	UNC Chapel Hill, USA
Guorong Wu	UNC Chapel Hill, USA
Horst Bischof	TU Graz, Austria
Jan Margeta	Inria, France
Jürgen Gall	Bonn University, Germany
Kayhan Batmanghelich	MIT, USA
Kilian Pohl	Stanford University, USA

Koen Leemput	Harvard Medical School, USA
Le Lu	NIH, USA
Luping Zhou	University of Wollongong, Australia
Michael Wels	Siemens Healthcare, Germany
Milan Sonka	University of Iowa, USA
Nassir Navab	TU Munich, Germany
Ruogu Fang	Florida International University, USA
Tom Vercauteren	University College London, UK
Vasileios Zografos	TU Munich, Germany
Yang Song	University of Sydney, Australia
Yefeng Zheng	Siemens Corporate Research, USA
Yong Xia	Northwestern Polytechnical University, China
Yue Gao	National University of Singapore, Singapore

Program Committee BAMBI 2016

Bennett Landeman	Vanderbilt University, USA
Carole Sudre	UCL, UK
Dongjin Kwon	SRI International, USA
Eugenio Iglesias	UCL, UK
Guido Gerig	NYU, USA
Marco Lorenzi	UCL, UK
Mattias Heinrich	University of Lübeck, Germany
Maxime Taquet	Harvard Medical School, USA
Monica Enescu	University of Oxford, UK
Kayhan Batmanghelich	MIT, USA
Suyash Awate	IITB, India

Contents

BAMBI Workshop

MCV Workshop: Brain Imaging

Constructing Subject- and Disease-Specific Effect Maps: Application to Neurodegenerative Diseases

Ender Konukoglu[1]([✉]) and Ben Glocker[2]

[1] Computer Vision Laboratory, ETH Zurich, Zurich, Switzerland
ender.konukoglu@vision.ee.ethz.ch
[2] Biomedical Image Analysis Group, Imperial College London, London, UK
b.glocker@imperial.ac.uk

Abstract. Current statistical methods in neuroimaging identify effects of neurodegenerative diseases on the brain structure by detecting group differences. Results are detailed maps showing population-wide effects. Although useful for better understanding the disease, these maps provide little subject-specific information. Furthermore, since group assignments have to be known prior to analysis, resulting maps have limited diagnostic value for new subjects. This article proposes a method to construct subject- and disease-specific effect maps prior to diagnosis. The method combines techniques from binary classification and image restoration to identify the effects of a disease of interest on the measurements. Experimental evaluation is carried out with synthetically generated data and real data selected from the ADNI cohort. Results demonstrate the capability of the proposed method in generating subject-specific effect maps.

1 Introduction

Statistical analysis of neuroimaging data has been instrumental in identifying structural variations of the human brain due to neurodegenerative diseases. Methods that can process high-dimensional image-based measurements allow constructing detailed volumetric [1] and surface maps [2,3] that highlight disease-affected areas in the brain. Such disease-effect maps have been studied for various neurodegenerative conditions in the literature [4–6]. These maps provide insights into conditions' characteristics and progression, guide histopathological studies and help developing image-based biomarkers.

Although immensely useful, current statistical methods that identify disease-specific effect-maps compute population-wide maps but they cannot compute *diagnostic subject-specific maps* that highlight disease-affected areas specific to a given subject prior to diagnosis. Inference-based models, whether univariate [1] or multivariate [7,8], detect condition-related differences in image-based measurements between two groups of subjects, one composed of patients and the other composed of controls. Detected differences are "averages" across the population and methods need diagnostic information for all subjects. Predictive

© Springer International Publishing AG 2017
H. Müller et al. (Eds.): MCV/BAMBI 2016, LNCS 10081, pp. 3–13, 2017.
DOI: 10.1007/978-3-319-61188-4_1

modeling approaches use machine-learning tools to identify measurements that are highly informative for diagnosing the condition [9–12]. Although the predictions of diagnosis are prospective, the identified areas are not and they are still population-wide.

Outlier detection is currently the only alternative for constructing maps that are subject-specific. Methods estimate normative (univariate or multivariate) distributions from a population consisting only of controls. The measurements of the subject under-investigation is then compared to the respective normative distributions and outliers are identified. This approach has been applied to brain lesion [13–16] and recently to neurodegenerative diseases [17]. It is however difficult to use outlier detection in constructing *disease-specific maps* because the methods themselves are not disease-specific. Given a new image, outlier detection methods will identify all abnormalities without specificity with respect to a disease of interest.

Why is it important to be able to construct diagnostic subject- and disease-specific maps? There are numerous applications for such a tool. First, it would enable studying variations of conditions' effects across the population to identify subgroups within the patients [18] and develop biomarkers of progression. Second, such maps would help analyzing cases where machine-learning tools fail, which would facilitate model improvements and possibly identifying misdiagnosis in the validation data. Lastly, subject- and disease-specific maps can complement "black-box" machine learning tools in their clinical application by providing reasonings and interpretation to the automatically generated decisions.

In this article we present a method to compute subject-specific and disease-specific diagnostic maps and show its application on neurodegenerative diseases. We focus on localized image-based measurements, such as widely used voxel-wise gray matter densities [1] and surface-based cortical thickness maps [3], as such measurements can be used to construct detailed maps of disease effects. The proposed method uses principles from binary classification and image denoising in a univariate setting. We present experiments evaluating the proposed technique on a synthetically generated dataset and on a cohort selected from the ADNI dataset. We compare the proposed tool to other methods including univariate general linear model [19] (GLM), support vector machines (SVM) [20] and random forests (RF) [21].

2   Method

Let us represent the image-based measurements extracted from a given subject's image with $\mathbf{f} = [f_1, ..., f_d] \in \mathbb{R}^d$. The goal of the method is to use $\mathbf{f}$ to construct a map $\mathbf{q} \in \{0,1\}^d$ that at each element indicates whether the corresponding measurement shows a condition effect (1) or not (0). To this end the method uses a training database $\{\mathbf{f}_n, y_n\}_{n=1,...,N}$, where y_n is a binary variable representing diagnostic information. We note that the method does not use the diagnostic information for the test image. We assume that all $\mathbf{f}_n$ and $\mathbf{f}$ are aligned and comparisons between corresponding elements are feasible[1].

---

[1] see http://www.fil.ion.ucl.ac.uk/spm/ or https://freesurfer.net to this end.

Intuition: The basis of the proposed method is that each element in **f** provides an independent probabilistic prediction on whether the subject has the condition, $y = 1$, or not, $y = 0$. This prediction, a simple element-wise classification result, indicates whether this element is affected by the condition of interest. The underlying intuition, and the novelty, of the proposed method is that element-wise classification results are viewed as noisy observations of underlying an "true" condition-effect map and the method aims to restore. To this end, there are two important components that can help the restoration process. First, prediction accuracy at each element can be estimated using the training dataset. Prediction estimate for an element indicates whether it shows consistent condition-effect throughout the population. This estimation can help correctly interpret (in other words down weigh) the predictions of measurements in a test image that does not show consistent condition-effect in the training set. Second, there is a topological relationship between the measurements in **f** when we consider surface meshes, images and volumes. Combining this with a smoothness assumption on the condition-effects on biological tissue, we utilize theory from Markov Random Fields and enforce consistency of estimated effect between neighboring measurements. Below we formulate this intuition and the two components.

We denote the independent element-wise predictions with $\mathbf{p} \in [0, 1]^d$ and model it with a Gaussian mixture model that has one component for each condition. We use equal priors for the components and compute the posterior probability with

$$p_j = p(y = 1|f_j) = \frac{\mathcal{N}(f_j; \mu_1^{(j)}, (\sigma_1^{(j)})^2)}{\sum_{g=0,1} \mathcal{N}(f_j; \mu_g^{(j)}, (\sigma_g^{(j)})^2)}, \quad j = 1, \ldots, d, \qquad (1)$$

where $\mu_{0,1}^{(j)}$ and $\sigma_{0,1}^{(j)}$ are the mean and standard deviations for the different groups empirically estimated from the training dataset. We model **p** as a noisy observation with logit-normal distribution where the noise is iid additive Gaussian noise in the logit domain, i.e. $\hat{\Phi}_j = \log(p_j/(1-p_j))$ and $\hat{\Phi}_j = \Phi_j + \epsilon$ where $\epsilon \sim \mathcal{N}(0, \sigma^2)$. In this formulation $\Phi = [\Phi_1, \ldots, \Phi_d]$ is the underlying noise-free disease-effect map we are aiming to restore. We further model the prior distribution of Φ with:

$$p(\Phi) = \frac{1}{Z} \exp\left\{ -\frac{1}{2} \left(\sum_j \kappa_j \Phi_j^2 + \lambda \sum_j \sum_{k \in N(j)} \frac{(\Phi_j - \Phi_k)^2}{(d\mu_j - d\mu_k)^2} \right) \right\},$$

where $N(j)$ is the neighborhood of the measurement j, $d\mu_j = \mu_1^{(j)}/\sigma_1^{(j)} - \mu_0^{(j)}/\sigma_0^{(j)}$, λ is the pairwise strength term, $\kappa_j = \tan(\eta_j \pi)$ where η_j is the prediction error rate of p_j (with thresholding at 0.5) estimated from the training dataset and max-limited at 0.5, and Z is the normalization constant. The role of the unary term is to enforce Φ_j to 0 for measurements that do not show predictive power in the training dataset. The $\tan(x)$ function is used because it is 0 when $x = 0$ and goes to ∞ as $x \to \pi/2$. The role of the pairwise term is to enforce consistency between neighboring measurements that show similar group-differences in the z-normalized GMM means. For localized image based measurements $N(j)$ is the set of immediate neighbors in the image domain or on the surface. For global measurements where neighborhood is not well-defined, such as volumes of anatomical structures, $N(j)$ can be an empty set or fully connected, however, here we only focus on the localized measurements.

Based on the prior and the observation model, the method computes the maximum-a-posteriori (MAP) estimate of Φ by solving

$$(\sigma^2 \kappa_j + 1)\Phi_j + \sigma^2 \lambda \sum_{k \in N(j)} \frac{\Phi_j - \Phi_k}{(d\mu_j - d\mu_k)^2} = \hat{\Phi}_j, \ j = 1, \cdots, d \qquad (2)$$

This system of linear equations can be solved efficiently even for large d using sparse routines for limited neighborhood sizes.

The MAP estimate Φ^* is a continuous valued map. In order to determine the $\mathbf{q}$ map, i.e. final regions that are affected by the condition, we would need to threshold Φ^*, i.e. $q_j = 1$ if $\Phi_j^* > \tau$ and 0 otherwise. The threshold τ could have been determined to maximize detection accuracy if the $\mathbf{q}_n$ maps were available for the training samples. Since this information is not available, instead, we assume that the control samples are subjects that should not have any disease-affected areas and $\mathbf{q}$ maps for these samples should be all zeros. Based on this we determine the τ threshold by limiting the false-positive-rate (FPR) on the control samples in the training dataset using

$$\tau = \min t, \ \text{such that}, \ \frac{1}{dN_{y=0}} \sum_{n \ \text{with} \ y_n=0} \sum_j \delta(\Phi_{n,j}^* > t) \leq \tau_{\text{FPR}}, \qquad (3)$$

where $N_{y=0}$ is the number of training control subjects and τ_{FPR} is the desired FPR limit. This optimization is one dimensional and can be solved efficiently with golden section search. Equation 3 allows the model to control the number of false positives over the entire set of measurements.

Estimating parameters with cross-validation and bootstrap: The parameters of the Gaussian mixture model, error rate estimates η and the threshold τ are estimated empirically using the training dataset. We implement a K-fold cross validation loop where at each fold Φ_n of control samples in the test partition are computed and τ is determined based on the cross-validation results. Within each fold we also use bootstrap sampling (sampling with replacement) on the training partition of the fold. $\mu_{0,1}$ and $\sigma_{0,1}$ are estimated by averaging bootstrap samples. η is estimated as the average of out-of-bag sample accuracies in each bootstrap experiment. This procedure avoids contamination between estimation of τ and the other parameters. For the σ parameter, we note that in Eq. 2 it is a multiplicative factor in front of κ_j and λ. Therefore, its effect on Φ will be through its interaction with the other terms. In order to reduce the number of tuning parameters of the model, in this work we set $\sigma = 1$.

Tuning parameters: λ and τ_{FPR} are the tuning parameters of the method. λ implements the strength of interaction between the neighboring measurements and it is related to the smoothness of the final maps. FPR is the amount of false positives a user is willing to accept in the resulting maps. Increase in FPR extends the detected areas at the expense of higher false detections.

Contributions: The novelties of the proposed method is the restoration formulation applied to element-wise binary classification results and the automatic determination of the threshold τ_{FPR} based on limiting false positive rates. To the best of our knowledge, this is the first work that produces subject and condition specific effect maps. It is also the first work that combines image restoration, binary classification and generalization accuracy estimation for this purpose. Lastly, this is the first work that predicts condition-affected areas in a diagnostic setting, i.e. without any information on the diagnosis of the test subject.

We note that **q** maps are subject-specific and they can vary drastically across subjects, which we demonstrate in Sect. 3. Furthermore, information they carry can be relevant for making subject-specific diagnosis.

3 Experiments

We evaluated the proposed method both with synthetically generated dataset and a cohort selected from the Alzheimer's Disease Neuroimaging Initiative (ADNI) dataset.

Synthetic Data: Ground truth information for disease-affected areas are often not available for in-vivo datasets. We generated a synthetic dataset that had two different types of disease effects with which we quantitatively analyze the retrieval and false positive rates of the proposed method. We generated 200 images, each of size 100×100, where 100 of them belong to the case (patient) group, with $y = 1$, and the other 100 to the control group. Images in the control group contained only stationary noise with spatial covariance and no underlying disease effect. We generated these images by assigning iid Gaussian noise at each pixel with 0 mean and $\sigma_n = 50$ standard deviation, and then blurring the image with a Gaussian kernel of standard deviation 2.5. Case images had the same noise but there were two different types of underlying disease effects, shown in Fig. 1. The effects shared the center white square but differed in the corner ones. The case group consisted of 50 images for each types of disease effects. We experimented with different effect-sizes, i.e. intensities of the squares, but in each experiment squares in the same image had the same effect-size. We generated the case images by adding blurred iid noise with σ_n to the images with white squares, where the blurring was done with the same Gaussian kernel as before. Examples of a control image and two case images of different types are shown in Fig. 1. The image-based measurements were simply taken as the image intensities.

We first applied GLM, RF and SVMs to identify population-wide disease-affected areas. For GLM we extracted p-value maps and corrected for multiple comparisons with Bonferroni's method. For both RF and SVM, we trained the methods with all the data and computed feature importances for RF and weights for SVM using scikit-learn package [22]. We converted importance values and

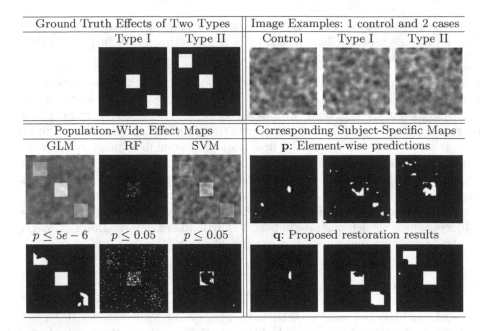

Fig. 1. Synthetic dataset visual results. LEFT: Two different types of disease effects were generated (top row). Second and third rows show group-wise identified areas by GLM, SVM and RF (second row: coefficients, third row: thresholded p-value maps). As can be seen in these images, population-wide results do not capture subject-specific effects. RIGHT: Top row shows three example images with noise std $\sigma_n = 50$ and underlying effect size $1.0 * \sigma_n$. Second row shows corresponding thresholded map based on element-wise predictions, i.e. $\mathbf{p}$ maps computed with Eq. 1, before the proposed restoration is applied. Third row shows the output of the proposed method $\mathbf{q}$ maps, which are restored versions of the element-wise predictions with Eq. 2 and thresholded using the value given by Eq. 3. Observe that the method indeed captures subject-specific disease effects. $\lambda = 0.5$ and $\tau_{\mathrm{FPR}} = 0.01$ for these results.

weights to p-values with permutation testing [9, 23] and thresholded the p-values manually. The results are shown in Fig. 1. We observe that all these methods detect population-wide disease-effects but the resulting maps do not provide subject-specific information.

We then tested the proposed method using 5-fold cross validation (CV). Parameters were estimated with an inner 5-fold CV loop as described in Sect. 2. In addition to $\mathbf{q}$ maps we also computed $\mathbf{p}$ maps that have independent element-wise predictions at each point before restoration. For $\mathbf{p}$ maps we also determined the optimal threshold by limiting FPR with Eq. 3. We repeated the experiment for different λ values, FPR thresholds 0.01 and 0.001, and five effect sizes $0.60\sigma_n$, $1.0\sigma_n$, $1.40\sigma_n$, $2.0\sigma_n$ and $3.0\sigma_n$.

Figure 1 shows visual examples of $\mathbf{q}$ and thresholded $\mathbf{p}$ maps obtained using $\lambda = 0.5$ and $\tau_{\mathrm{FPR}} = 0.01$. $\mathbf{q}$ maps show that the method detects the underlying subject-specific effects. Differences between $\mathbf{p}$ and $\mathbf{q}$ maps demonstrate the

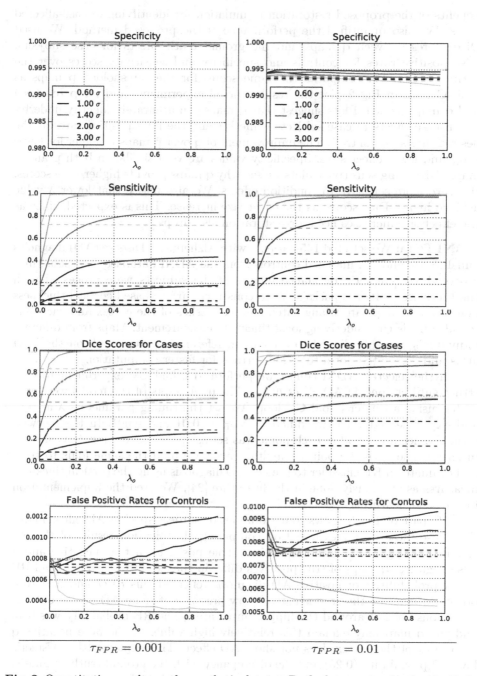

Fig. 2. Quantitative results on the synthetic dataset. Dashed curves are for thresholded **p** maps, i.e. measurement-wise binary classification results, and solid curves are for **q** maps, i.e. results of the proposed restoration method.

benefits of the proposed restoration formulation for identifying disease-affected areas. We also quantified the performance of the proposed method. We used Dice scores between q maps and the ground truth effects for case subjects, false positive rates for controls and specificity and sensitivity scores over the entire dataset. We computed the same scores for the thresholded p maps as well. Graphs in Fig. 2 plot the results for all experiments and for p (dashed) and q maps (solid). Plots suggest that q maps can accurately identify underlying disease effects in case subjects while keeping the false positive rates at the desired limits for controls. The improvement of q over p maps is higher for lower τ_{FPR} and lower effect sizes. Specificity values are very similar in both p and q maps. Observing sensitivity plots we see why q maps provide higher Dice scores: they are more sensitive to condition effects. We also notice that lower λ value achieve higher Dice scores as the effect size increase. This is expected, since as the effect-size increases need for restoration also drops.

ADNI Data: We selected 145 patients with Alzheimer's Disease (AD) diagnosis and 145 age and sex matched controls from the ADNI database. The structural T1-weighted magnetic resonance images of the subjects were processed with the Freesurfer software package [3] to construct surface-based cortical thickness maps. These maps are triangulated surface meshes of the cortex and each vertex also holds the underlying local thickness measurement. Maps from different individuals were all aligned to a common reference surface mesh on the MNI atlas and decimated down to 10242 vertices for faster computation.

On the selected ADNI cohort we performed 5-fold CV experiment to construct subject-specific AD-effect maps. The parameters of the model were estimated using an inner 5-fold CV loop. We set the tuning parameters λ as 0.15 and experimented with two different $\tau_{FPR} = 0.01$ and 0.001. In the pairwise term the neighborhood of each point was set as the set of vertices that share a mesh triangle with the point. Simultaneously, we used the same folds to train and evaluate an RF classifier to predict AD diagnosis using the cortical thickness measures as previously done in the literature [24]. We used the implementation in the scikit-learn package [22].

Left part of Fig. 3 shows four examples of subject-specific AD-effect maps. We chose these examples based on comparing classification results of the RF classifier and ground truth diagnosis: 2 true positives, a true negative and a false negative. q maps of true positives differ in the extent of the effect and RF based probabilities of positive AD diagnosis reflected this (0.77 and 0.91 top-down). q map for the true negative show presence of some AD effects but the detections are not around the hippocampal area. The RF probability was 0.46 and the q map may explain this relatively high value. In the false negative q map most of the cortex does not show AD effect. This explains RF classifier's low AD probability (0.25) and the discrepancy with the ground truth diagnosis.

At the right of Fig. 3 we show a frequency map of AD effect per vertex, where each vertex shows the portion of the patient cohort for which cortical thickness at that vertex showed AD effect in the q map. Not surprisingly, the pattern resembles previous group-analysis results for AD [25]. However, the crucial point

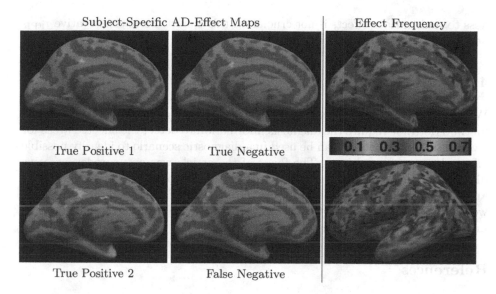

Fig. 3. Results on the ADNI dataset: Subject-specific effect maps of four subjects. Note the variation. Naming is based on comparing RF classification result and ground truth diagnosis. MIDDLE: Portion of patient cohort affected at each vertex.

is that the values correspond to number of patients not correlations. This makes this output much more interesting than correlations which cannot be trivially linked to concrete numbers. We note that most of the areas that are believed to be AD-related only show effect in less than 50% of the patient cohort.

Lastly, the proposed method is univariate in essence. Each measurement performs an independent prediction and MAP formulation "denoises" these predictions. This approach would be blind to multivariate interactions if they exist. To quantify the effect of this blindness in the ADNI cohort, we evaluated the value of **q** maps for AD versus control classification. We used 10 randomly shuffled 5-fold cross validation experiments to train and evaluate an RF classifier using thickness measures and **q** maps. Classification accuracies (ACC) and area-under-the-curve (AUC) scores are given in the Table 1. Results suggest that **q** maps retain the predictive information in the thickness measurements and blind-

Table 1. Classification results: AD versus control classification using thickness measurements and **q** maps with Random Forest. **q** maps retain the information in thickness measures.

	Cortical thickness	$\mathbf{q} \ @ \ \tau_{FPR} = 0.01$	$\mathbf{q} \ @ \ \tau_{FPR} = 0.001$
ACC	0.827 ± 0.007	0.833 ± 0.009	0.810 ± 0.010
AUC	0.908 ± 0.002	0.891 ± 0.004	0.858 ± 0.010

ness to multivariate effects is not crucial for this cohort. More conservative τ_{FPR} decreased prediction accuracies of q maps.

4 Conclusions

We proposed a method for constructing subject-specific disease-effect maps. The method does not require the diagnosis information to detect the affected areas for a given subject. Hence, it can be used in a diagnostic scenario to identify possible affected areas of a subjects. The focus of the article was on neurodegenerative diseases and in particular on AD. However, the method is generic enough to be applied to other disorders of the brain and possibly of other body parts. Future work focuses on extending the method to multivariate interactions and global image-based measurements.

References

1. Ashburner, J., Friston, K.J.: Why voxel-based morphometry should be used. Neuroimage **14**(6), 1238–1243 (2001)
2. Greve, D.N.: An absolute beginner's guide to surface-and voxel-based morphometric analysis. Proc. Intl. Soc. Mag. Reson. Med. **19**, 33 (2011)
3. Fischl, B.: Freesurfer. Neuroimage **62**(2), 774–781 (2012)
4. Thompson, P.M., et al.: Cortical change in Alzheimer's disease detected with a disease-specific population-based brain atlas. Cereb. Cortex **11**(1), 1–16 (2001)
5. Rosas, H., et al.: Regional and progressive thinning of the cortical ribbon in huntington's disease. Neurology **58**(5), 695–701 (2002)
6. Burton, E.J., et al.: Cerebral atrophy in Parkinson's disease with and without dementia: a comparison with Alzheimer's disease, dementia with lewy bodies and controls. Brain **127**(4), 791–800 (2004)
7. Krishnan, A., et al.: Partial least squares (PLS) methods for neuroimaging: a tutorial and review. Neuroimage **56**(2), 455–475 (2011)
8. Worsley, K.J., et al.: Characterizing the response of PET and fMRI data using multivariate linear models. Neuroimage **6**(4), 305–319 (1997)
9. Gaonkar, B., Davatzikos, C.: Analytic estimation of statistical significance maps for support vector machine based multi-variate image analysis and classification. Neuroimage **78**, 270–283 (2013)
10. Mwangi, B., Tian, T.S., Soares, J.C.: A review of feature reduction techniques in neuroimaging. Neuroinformatics **12**(2), 229–244 (2014)
11. Rahim, M., Thirion, B., Abraham, A., Eickenberg, M., Dohmatob, E., Comtat, C., Varoquaux, G.: Integrating multimodal priors in predictive models for the functional characterization of Alzheimer's disease. In: Navab, N., Hornegger, J., Wells, W.M., Frangi, A.F. (eds.) MICCAI 2015. LNCS, vol. 9349, pp. 207–214. Springer, Cham (2015). doi:10.1007/978-3-319-24553-9_26
12. Ganz, M., et al.: Relevant feature set estimation with a knock-out strategy and random forests. Neuroimage **122**, 131–148 (2015)
13. Maumet, C., Maurel, P., Ferré, J.C., Barillot, C.: An a contrario approach for the detection of patient-specific brain perfusion abnormalities with arterial spin labelling. Neuroimage **134**, 424–433 (2016)

14. Tomas-Fernandez, X., Warfield, S.K.: A model of population and subject (MOPS) intensities with application to multiple sclerosis lesion segmentation. IEEE Trans. Med. Imaging **34**(6), 1349–1361 (2015)
15. Van Leemput, K., Maes, F., Vandermeulen, D., Colchester, A., Suetens, P.: Automated segmentation of multiple sclerosis lesions by model outlier detection. IEEE Trans. Med. Imaging **20**(8), 677–688 (2001)
16. Prastawa, M.: A brain tumor segmentation framework based on outlier detection*1. Med. Image Anal. **8**(3), 275–283 (2004)
17. Zeng, K., Erus, G., Sotiras, A., Shinohara, R.T., Davatzikos, C.: Abnormality detection via iterative deformable registration and basis-pursuit decomposition. IEEE Trans. Med. Imaging **PP**(99), 1 (2016)
18. Iqbal, K.: Subgroups of Alzheimer's disease based on cerebrospinal fluid molecular markers. Ann. Neurol. **58**(5), 748–757 (2005)
19. Kiebel, S., Holmes, P.: The General Linear Model. Academic Press, London (2003)
20. Cortes, C., Vapnik, V.: Support-vector networks. Mach. Learn. **20**(3), 273–297 (1995)
21. Breiman, L.: Random forests. Mach. Learn. **45**(1), 5–32 (2001)
22. Pedregosa, F., et al.: Scikit-learn: machine learning in Python. J. Mach. Learn. Res. **12**, 2825–2830 (2011)
23. Good, P.I.: Permutation, Parametric and Bootstrap Tests of Hypotheses. Springer, Heidelberg (2005)
24. Sabuncu, M.R., Konukoglu, E.: Clinical prediction from structural brain MRI scans: a large-scale empirical study. Neuroinformatics **13**(1), 31–46 (2015)
25. Dickerson, B.C., et al.: The cortical signature of alzheimer's disease: regionally specific cortical thinning relates to symptom severity in very mild to mild ad dementia and is detectable in asymptomatic amyloid positive individuals. Cereb. Cortex **19**(3), 497–510 (2009)

BigBrain: Automated Cortical Parcellation and Comparison with Existing Brain Atlases

Marc Fournier$^{(\boxtimes)}$, Lindsay B. Lewis, and Alan C. Evans

Brain Imaging Centre, Montreal Neurological Institute,
McGill University, Montreal, Canada
{marc.fournier2,lindsay.lewis,alan.evans}@mcgill.ca

Abstract. Most available 3D human brain atlases provide information only at a macroscopic level, while 2D atlases are often at a microscopic level but lack 3D integration. A 3D atlas defined upon fine-grain anatomical detail of cortical layers and cells is necessary to fully understand neurobiological processes. "BigBrain," a high-resolution 3D model of a human brain at nearly cellular resolution, was released in 2013. This unique dataset enables the extraction of microscopic data for utilization in brain mapping, modeling and simulation. We propose an automated 3D cortical parcellation of the BigBrain volume into functionally-meaningful areas in order to create a modern high-resolution 3D cytoarchitectural atlas that will complement existing brain atlases. We use a distance metrics-based framework for BigBrain parcellation, and perform comparative analyses of our results with existing atlases (Brodmann and JuBrain atlases). This work has immediate application in teaching, neurosurgery, cognitive neuroscience, and imaging-based brain mapping.

Keywords: Brain atlases · Cortical cytoarchitecture · Segmentation and parcellation · Brain mapping · Image registration · Computational neuroscience

1 Introduction

Reference brains in human brain mapping are indispensable tools, enabling integration of multimodal data into a common framework. However, most presently available human brain atlases do not provide information beyond the macroscopic level. Fine-grain anatomical resolution of cortical layers, columns, microcircuits, and cells is necessary to fully understand neurobiological processes.

In 2013 "BigBrain" [1], a high-resolution digital 3D model of a human brain reconstructed from 7,404 histological sections at a nearly cellular isotropic resolution of 20 μm, was created. The dataset is publicly available and includes 3D tissue classification as well as cortical surface extraction.

In this paper, we propose a 3D automated cortical parcellation of the BigBrain volume into functionally-meaningful areas, which should complement existing brain atlases such as the Brodmann atlas [2] and JuBrain atlas [3]. Although the 3D Brodmann atlas is widely used in neuroimaging, it is not a gold standard, neither validated

© Springer International Publishing AG 2017
H. Müller et al. (Eds.): MCV/BAMBI 2016, LNCS 10081, pp. 14–25, 2017.
DOI: 10.1007/978-3-319-61188-4_2

nor based on robust cytoarchitectural boundaries. The JuBrain atlas is, like our current work, a high resolution cytoarchitectural atlas; however it consists of an initial 2D partial manual segmentation prior to its reconstruction in 3D. The 2D manual segmentation is guided by algorithms which utilize a local gray level index [4]. Due to the intensive manual nature of this segmentation, there are many areas of the JuBrain atlas that are not yet complete.

Previous work on 3D automated methods to parcellate brain images has been done using different imaging modalities of standard resolution such as MRI [5], fMRI [6], DTI [7] and SPECT [8]. These methods have been designed to operate at the macroscopic scale and most of them [5, 7, 8] propose parcellation schemes based on Mahalanobis and Euclidean distance metrics. While our parcellation framework is designed to operate on cytoarchitecture at the microscopic scale, it is similarly based on distance metrics including Mahalanobis and Euclidean distances.

Although parcellation of brain cytoarchitectural histology data has been addressed previously, in most cases the parcellation is done on 2D sections, and only afterwards are the segmented structures reconstructed in 3D [9, 10]. This approach restricts the definition of cytoarchitectural boundaries to two dimensions, on a single section at a time. Our new method overcomes this restriction and allows the detection of boundaries in 3D. Moreover, in contrast to previous work where cytoarchitectural boundaries are typically manually delineated by experts, our proposed method is automated.

It should be noted that recent work has also been done on the manual segmentation of the BigBrain volume in specific areas such as substructures of basal ganglia [11], with immediate clinical applications in neurosurgery [12]. The new cytoarchitectural brain atlas that we are currently proposing (again, which is automated and extends across the entire cortex) will be additionally useful for many applications in clinical and fundamental brain research, in all areas where the ubiquitous 3D Brodmann atlas is used.

The nature of the BigBrain dataset is unique. On the one hand, previous automated parcellation methods proposed for macroscopic MR images were not designed to assess cytoarchitectural boundaries. On the other hand, manual and semi-automated methods proposed to parcellate 2D cellular-level cytoarchitectural sections are not suited for the 3D volume of the BigBrain at near-cellular resolution. Therefore, the parcellation method described in this paper is especially designed for the BigBrain and inspired from previous work in both fields.

Derived from the BigBrain dataset, the goal of the proposed atlas is therefore two-fold; (1) to provide a much more modern, high level of resolution, and (2) to be defined upon cytoarchitectural boundaries truly detected in 3D. In order to compare our parcellation of the BigBrain to other existing atlases, we used the method described in [13], which proposes a comprehensive set of measures for quantitative comparison of anatomical parcellations of brain atlases. This method allows the evaluation of atlases with differing numbers of regions. It is an interesting feature for the analysis of our results that the generated parcellations are likely to have different numbers of final regions. To perform our analysis, we selected a subset of the measures proposed in that method.

2   Materials and Methods

2.1   Material: BigBrain Volume, Brodmann and JuBrain Atlases

The BigBrain volume is available in various file formats and reference spaces (https://bigbrain.loris.ca). In this work, in order to avoid any distortion that may be introduced by additional processes such as registration into stereotaxic space, we used the 2015 version of the BigBrain 3D reconstructed volume in its native histological space. Such distortion could otherwise have a negative impact on parcellation results. To define the cortical mantle, which consists of voxels labeled as gray matter, we used the available 3D classified volume image and gray and white matter surfaces, extracted at 200 μm.

Additionally, we used the 3D Brodmann atlas provided with MRIcron software (available at http://www.mccauslandcenter.sc.edu/mricro/mricron). The atlas was registered to the BigBrain volume in order to compare our parcellations of the BigBrain to the projected Brodmann areas. We focused our work on the left hemisphere of the brain since the Brodmann atlas was initially defined on the left hemisphere. The right hemisphere of the atlas is a symmetric copy of the left.

For specific regions such as visual cortex, we also chose to compare our parcellation results with the JuBrain atlas (available at http://www.fz-juelich.de/inm/inm-1/EN/Forschung/JuBrain/Jubrain_Webtools/Jubrain_Webtools_node.html). The ongoing construction of this atlas is performed using a semi-automated parcellation method [4] previously introduced to assist experts in delineation of cytoarchitectural boundaries upon 2D slices. This method uses distance metrics to capture differences between cytoarchitectural profiles.

We adapted this method for the BigBrain dataset, but because this method was designed to operate at a cellular resolution of 1 μm, we failed to obtain significant parcellations. Image processing tools provided by this method count individual cell bodies in a region of interest. At the resolution of the BigBrain (20 μm), individual cells are not visible; therefore this method was not appropriate to achieve our goal.

2.2   Methods: Multilevel Parcellations Algorithm Approach (Overview)

Our analysis consisted of an initialization phase followed by a tri-level parcellation approach (Fig. 1). At the initialization phase, described in Sect. 2.3 below, initial profiles (163,842 3D bars) were defined and dropped across the cortical mantle, maximizing coverage while avoiding overlap. Using a Scale-Invariant Feature Transform (SIFT) algorithm these initial profiles were triaged down to 1,071 starting profiles that represented the maximally homogenous centers within groups of profiles exhibiting similar information (while being maximally distant from borders of profiles exhibiting different information). The tri-level parcellation approach is based on a distance metric framework, which is described in Sect. 2.4 below.

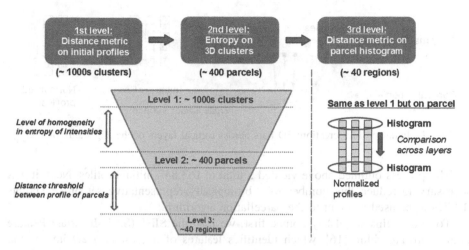

Fig. 1. Multilevel parcellation algorithm divided into three levels from fine to coarse.

At the first level of parcellation, described in Sect. 2.5 below, distances between the starting profiles and their neighbors were computed. Similar neighboring profiles were collapsed together to form 3D clusters in a data-driven, region-growing process which yielded 1,071 clusters. The second (intermediate) level of parcellation, described in Sect. 2.6 below, was introduced in order to bridge the gap between the first and third levels of parcellation. The entropy of the previously obtained 3D clusters was used to merge similar ones, reducing these 1,071 clusters to ~400 parcels (entropy thresholds were user-defined and adjusted to target a number that is one order of magnitude higher than the final target in the third level). At the third level of parcellation, described in Sect. 2.7 below, distance metrics were again employed, this time onto the histograms of the previously obtained ~400 parcels in order to reduce them to ~40 final regions (distance metric thresholds were also user-defined and adjusted to target a comparable number of regions as the Brodmann atlas).

2.3 Methods: Initial Profiles and Algorithm Starting Points (Initialization)

First, initial profiles were created over the entire cortical mantle of the BigBrain. A profile is a column which begins with a voxel on the gray matter surface, transversing down through the cortical layers in the direction of the gray matter surface normal vector, and ends with a voxel on the white matter surface, as schematized in Fig. 2. By applying the Laplace equation as proposed in [14], we determined that using a 3D 18-connected neighborhood for voxels along the path would provide maximum density of profiles without overlap. Next, in order to assure robustness of profiles to effects of curvature on layer compression, we used an equivolumic cortical depth model [15]. Finally, all profiles were normalized to straight vectors of identical length, with values corresponding to voxel intensities across cortical layers.

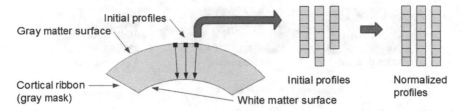

Fig. 2. Initial profiles creation: 3D bars across cortical layers of the BigBrain volume.

The process outlined above yielded a total of 163,842 initial profiles. Next, it was necessary to reduce this number to a biologically representative set of key points (1,071) to be used as input to the parcellation algorithm.

To choose this set of key points, first, we used the SIFT (Scale-Invariant Feature Transform) algorithm [16], which identifies features of interest in a 2D image, and adapted it to determine 3D key points of interest. We used Eq. (1) to compute in 3D the gradient amplitude and angles of each voxel.

$$Amp = \sqrt{G_x^2 + G_y^2 + G_z^2}; \ \theta = a\tan\left(\frac{G_y}{G_x}\right); \ \varphi = a\tan\left(\frac{G_z}{\sqrt{G_x^2 + G_y^2}}\right) \tag{1}$$

Then we constructed an orientation histogram as proposed in [17] for the 3D neighborhood around a given interest point by dividing θ and ϕ into bins of equal size. While working in 3D, it was also necessary to normalize the values added to each bin by the area of the bin as described in [18]. This corresponds to the solid angle Ω computed using Eq. (2). The values added to the histogram were computed using Eq. (3) where (x_n, y_n, z_n) represented the location of the voxel being added to the histogram of the interest point.

$$\Omega = \int_{\varphi}^{\varphi + \Delta\varphi} \int_{\theta}^{\theta + \Delta\theta} \sin\theta \ d\theta \ d\varphi = \Delta\varphi[\cos\theta - \cos(\theta + \Delta\theta)] \tag{2}$$

$$hist = \frac{1}{\Omega} Amp(x_n, y_n, z_n) e^{-\left[\frac{(x-x_n)^2 + (y-y_n)^2 + (z-z_n)^2}{2\sigma^2}\right]} \tag{3}$$

In this manner, we were able to obtain preliminary key points that were more likely to be close to the parcels' borders (where information was most heterogeneous).

Second, we performed an additional step to shift those key points away from each border and instead more centrally, toward profiles exhibiting maximally homogeneous information. Accordingly, our starting points would be in the presumed center of a given region. To accomplish this, we tessellated the key points by generating a tetrahedral mesh based on a 3D Delaunay triangulation algorithm [19]. Then, we computed its dual mesh (also known as the Voronoi diagram). The set of voxels located in the center of the tetrahedrons (corresponding to the Voronoi diagram vertices) were used as the starting points of our parcellation algorithm.

2.4 Methods: Distance Metrics Definitions (Used at First and Third Levels)

Our parcellation algorithm is based upon measurements of distance metrics, assessed between initial profiles (first level) and then again between 3D parcels (third level). Distance metrics serve as similarity criteria, comparing the (dis)similarity of intensity properties. In this analysis, we tested a subset of the distance metrics surveyed in [20] in order to identify the most suitable metric for our parcellation task. Our goal was to select those metrics that were most informative about different, complementary features, while disregarding those that were redundantly informative about similar features. The distance metrics tested are listed in Table 1.

Table 1. List of distance metrics used in the parcellation algorithm

City block	$d(x,y) = \sum_{i=1}^{n} \lvert x_i - y_i \rvert$	Canberra	$d(x,y) = \sum_{i=1}^{n} \frac{\lvert x_i - y_i \rvert}{\lvert x_i + y_i \rvert}$
Euclidean	$d(x,y) = \sqrt{\sum_{i=1}^{n} (x_i - y_i)^2}$	Squared chord	$d(x,y) = \sum_{i=1}^{n} \left(\sqrt{x_i} - \sqrt{y_i} \right)^2$
Minkowski	$d(x,y) = \left(\sum_{i=1}^{n} \lvert x_i - y_i \rvert^p \right)^{1/p}$	Squared Chi	$d(x,y) = \sqrt{\sum_{i=1}^{n} \frac{(x_i - y_i)^2}{\lvert x_i + y_i \rvert}}$

In the first column of Table 1, we selected widely used distances of the same L_p family, with City block and Euclidean distances being particular cases of the Minkowski distance when $p = 1$ and $p = 2$, respectively. For Minkowski distance, we selected $p = 3$ in order to obtain better results. In the second column of Table 1, we selected other distances among the most used in their respective families: Canberra distance belongs to L_1 family, Squared chord to *Fidelity* family, and Squared Chi to *Squared L_2* family. In addition to the six Table 1 distance metrics that we obtained from [20], we additionally tested the Mahalanobis distance [21], defined by Eq. (4).

$$d(x,y) = \sqrt{(x-y)^T S^{-1}(x-y)} \ where : S = covariance \ matrix \qquad (4)$$

It is worth noting that if the elements of x and y are independents, then the covariance matrix will be the identity one, and in that case the Mahalanobis distance would be equal to the Euclidean distance. In two dimensions, equal distances from a center point are represented by circles for the Euclidean distance, and for the Mahalanobis distance they are represented by ellipses.

2.5 Methods: Distance Metrics (First Level)

For each of the seven distance metrics selected, the following procedure (schematized in Fig. 1) was independently performed. As already described, the initialization phase considered all initial profiles (163,842), using the adapted 3D SIFT algorithm in order to select the starting profiles (1,071).

Next, distances between starting profiles and their neighbors were computed. Neighboring profiles with distances under a predefined threshold were labeled and collapsed together to form 3D clusters. In a region-growing process, the scope moved from starting profiles to the labeled neighbor ones. Distances were then computed between labeled profiles and their nearest neighbors. This process terminated when all of the initial profiles had ultimately been assigned to an existing cluster. The distance threshold was initially set at a low value. If initial profiles remained unlabeled, the process iterated with an increased threshold until all profiles belonged to a cluster.

Of additional interest, this highly detailed parcellation (1,071 clusters) may be advantageously combined with recently emerging new atlases at high-resolution such as [22], which defines ~ 900 neuroanatomically precise subdivisions based on genomic transcriptome distributions of the brain.

2.6   Methods: Entropy Measurements (Second Level)

In the second level of parcellation, using entropy measurements, the 1,071 3D clusters were input as seeds to grow ~ 400 parcels. This intermediate level of parcellation was introduced in order to bridge the gap between the first and third level. In practice, this is useful to target a specific number of final regions with unit increment. Our entropy measurement [23] was defined by Eq. (5).

$$E(p(x)) = \sum_{x \in X} p(x) \log(p(x)) \, where : p(x) = histogram \, of \, x \qquad (5)$$

By definition this measure is not a metric because it does not satisfy some of the metric conditions such as symmetry and triangle inequality. Entropy is a statistical measure used to characterize the texture of our clusters obtained after the first level of parcellation. It gives a quantitative appreciation of homogeneity of a cluster in terms of intensities of its voxels. In order to compute the entropy measurement, we used 256 bins to construct the histogram counts of the clusters.

If two neighboring clusters exhibited similar entropy, they were regrouped together as a parcel, and the algorithm continued moving outward. If not, the algorithm stopped and it was defined as an edge or boundary of the parcel. The level of similarity required to merge clusters was set in such a way to obtain a number of parcels which is an order of magnitude higher than the number of final regions targeted. As shown in Fig. 1, since we were ultimately targeting close to 40 final regions for comparison with Brodmann areas (41 in the atlas used), the intermediate number was set to ~ 400 parcels.

2.7   Methods: Distance Metrics (Third Level)

At the third level of parcellation, histograms were constructed to characterize the distribution of the intensities of voxels across cortical layers in all previously obtained parcels (~ 400). Then, the same distance metric (used on single voxels of initial profiles at first level, described above in Sect. 2.5) was used in a similar way on the histograms of parcels. Here, the distance threshold between neighbor parcels was set to obtain the targeted number of final regions (~ 40).

3 Results

The proposed parcellation pipeline was processed with each metric. Results were selected based upon global similarity of parcellations in comparison to the Brodmann atlas, using a similarity index value yielded by a region-level concordance analysis proposed in [13]. The obtained results do not necessarily have exactly 41 regions; rather, the similarity index was used to target the best matches compared to Brodmann areas. The Mahalanobis distance metric obtained the highest similarity index score, and was therefore identified as the metric to best map the Brodmann parcellation scheme onto the BigBrain volume. Accordingly, its similarity index was used to normalize the similarity index of all other metrics in order to compare their results. Figure 3 shows the normalized indices and the number of regions for each metric result.

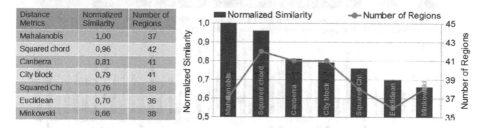

Distance Metrics	Normalized Similarity	Number of Regions
Mahalanobis	1,00	37
Squared chord	0,96	42
Canberra	0,81	41
City block	0,79	41
Squared Chi	0,76	38
Euclidean	0,70	36
Minkowski	0,66	38

Fig. 3. Evaluation of the distance metrics tested based on their similarity indices.

In Fig. 3, the metrics are ranked in decreasing order of similarity index. The second one in line is the Squared chord metric, which is very close to the Mahalanobis metric, and thus does not provide substantially different information. Both have different numbers of regions which do not exactly correspond to the number of Brodmann areas. The average number of regions for all metrics is 39, which is two regions less than the Brodmann atlas. The Canberra and City block metrics have 41 regions (same as the Brodmann atlas) and both have very similar indices, ranked third and fourth.

Figure 4 shows the parcellation result of the Mahalanobis metric, which was found to be the most similar to the Brodmann atlas based on the previous analysis. Figure 4(a) shows the Brodmann areas registered to the BigBrain left hemisphere, while Fig. 4(b) shows the Mahalanobis parcellation result. Both color codes are similar but they do not exactly match since the number of regions/areas are not the same. Figure 4(c) shows a quantitative analysis of volume concordance between Brodmann areas and our parcellation results. Mutual overlapping volume distribution is quantified between our result and the Brodmann atlas.

In Fig. 4(c), the blue columns show the fraction of the volume of a Brodmann area which is overlapped by the BigBrain parcellation region covering most of that area's volume. Likewise, the orange columns show the fraction of the volume of the BigBrain parcellation region (previously identified) which is overlapped by that same Brodmann

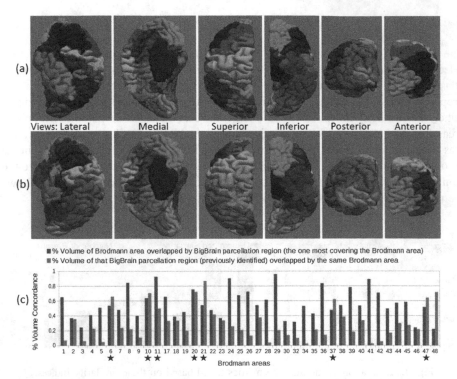

Fig. 4. Comparison of BigBrain parcellation with Brodmann atlas using Mahalanobis distance. (a) BigBrain left hemisphere with Brodmann areas. (b) BigBrain parcellation results using color coding similar to Brodmann areas in (a) to highlight concordance. (c) Chart of concordance between Brodmann areas and BigBrain parcellation regions. (Color figure online)

area. If a perfect match were to be attained for a specific Brodmann area, the value of both blue and orange columns for that area would be 1. The stars below selected Brodmann areas denote areas with high concordance, represented by higher values in both (blue and orange) columns.

Figure 5 shows (a) Mahalanobis and (b) Canberra results compared to JuBrain atlas in the visual cortex (Squared Chord was omitted because it demonstrated high similarity to Mahalanobis). These parcellations have been adapted by targeting a higher number of final regions in order to match the level of detail of the JuBrain segmentation in the visual cortex. In Fig. 5, the numbered arrows designate boundaries successfully detected by the parcellation algorithm compared to JuBrain areas, while lettered circles designate where the distance metrics have failed to detect some JuBrain areas.

This qualitative analysis highlights the complementarity of the distance metric results. For example, both failures with Mahalanobis (circles A and B, Fig. 5(a)) were successfully detected with Canberra (arrows 1 and 2, Fig. 5(b)) and inversely the failure with Canberra (circle A, Fig. 5(b)) was successfully detected with Mahalanobis (arrow 2, Fig. 5(a)). This observation demonstrates that, according to the JuBrain atlas, combining these two metrics may lead to a better parcellation. Ongoing work focuses on automated linear combination of metrics in order to optimize the results.

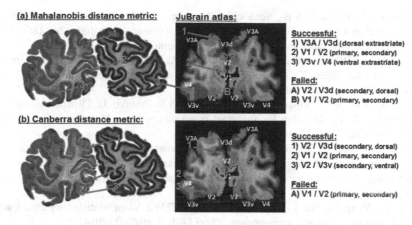

Fig. 5. Comparison of BigBrain parcellation with JuBrain atlas with focus on the visual cortex. (a) Mahalanobis distance compared to JuBrain. (b) Canberra distance compared to JuBrain.

4 Conclusion

We have proposed an automated parcellation of the BigBrain volume in order to provide a unique high-resolution modern cytoarchitectural 3D atlas. This work has immediate value across a broad range of applications, including teaching, neurosurgery, cognitive neuroscience, and imaging-based brain mapping. Our parcellation framework is based upon distance metrics, and we performed comparative analyses of our results with existing brain atlases. Future work will include refinement of the parcellation using consensus between complementary distance metrics, and validation of results from a functional neuroanatomy perspective.

Acknowledgements. We acknowledge funding support from the Canadian Institutes of Health Research (CIHR) and from Canada's Advanced Research and Innovation Network (CANARIE). We thank Compute Canada for continued support accessing the Compute Canada HPC grid through the CBRAIN software portal. We also thank Svenja Caspers for helpful discussion and providing expertise in neuroanatomy as well as Katrin Amunts and Karl Zilles from the Jülich Research Centre in Germany.

References

1. Amunts, K., Lepage, C., Borgeat, L., Mohlberg, H., Dickscheid, T., Rousseau, M.E., Bludau, S., Bazin, P.L., Lewis, L.B., Oros-Peusquens, A.M., Shah, N.J., Lippert, T., Zilles, K., Evans, A.C.: BigBrain: an ultrahigh-resolution 3D human brain model. Science **340**, 1472–1475 (2013)
2. Brodmann, K.: Vergleichende Lokalisationslehre der Grosshirnrinde. Johann Ambrosius Bart, Leipzig (1909)

3. Mohlberg, H., Eickhoff, S.B., Schleicher, A., Zilles, K., Amunts, K.: A new processing pipeline and release of cytoarchitectonic probabilistic maps – JuBrain. In: 18th Annual Meeting of the Organization for Human Brain Mapping, Beijing, China (2012)
4. Schleicher, A., Palomero-Gallagher, N., Morosan, P., Eickhoff, S.B., Kowalski, T., de Vos, K., Amunts, K., Zilles, K.: Quantitative architectural analysis: a new approach to cortical mapping. Anatomy Embryol. 210, 373–386 (2005)
5. Hemanth, D.J., Selva Vijila, C.K., Selvakumar, A.I., Anitha, J.: Distance metric-based time-efficient fuzzy algorithm for abnormal magnetic resonance brain image segmentation. Neural Comput. Appl. 22, 1013–1022 (2013)
6. Sanchez-Panchuelo, R.M., Besle, J., Beckett, A., Bowtell, R., Schluppeck, D., Francis, S.: Within-digit functional parcellation of brodmann areas of the human primary somatosensory cortex using functional magnetic resonance imaging at 7 tesla. J. Neurosci. 32, 15815–15822 (2012)
7. Kong, Y., Wang, D., Shi, L., Hui, S.C.N., Chu, W.C.W.: Adaptive distance metric learning for diffusion tensor image segmentation. PLoS ONE 9, e92069 (2014)
8. Chaves, R., Ramírez, J., Górriz, J.M., Illán, I., Segovia, F., Olivares, A.: Effective diagnosis of alzheimer's disease by means of distance metric learning and random forest. In: Ferrández, J.M., Álvarez Sánchez, J.R., Paz, F., Toledo, F.J. (eds.) IWINAC 2011. LNCS, vol. 6687, pp. 59–67. Springer, Heidelberg (2011). doi:10.1007/978-3-642-21326-7_7
9. Uylingsa, H.B.M., Sanz-Arigita, E.J., de Vos, K., Pool, C.W., Evers, P., Rajkowska, G.: 3-D cytoarchitectonic parcellation of human orbitofrontal cortex correlation with postmortem MRI. Psychiatry Res. Neuroimaging 183, 1–20 (2010)
10. Caspers, S., Geyer, S., Schleicher, A., Mohlberg, H., Amunts, K., Zilles, K.: The human inferior parietal cortex: cytoarchitectonic parcellation and interindividual variability. NeuroImage 33, 430–448 (2006)
11. Altinkaya, A., Lepage, C., Lewis, L.B., Toussaint, P.J., Amunts, K., Zilles, K., Evans, A.C., Sadikot, A.F.: Ultrahigh resolution 3-d volumetric atlas of the human basal ganglia. In: 21st Annual Meeting of the Organization for Human Brain Mapping, Honolulu, USA (2015)
12. Altinkaya, A., Lepage, C., Ferreira, M., Pike, G.B., Evans, A.C., Sadikot A.F.: Registration of the bigbrain basal ganglia atlas to MNI space with surgical applications. In: 21st Annual Meeting of the Organization for Human Brain Mapping, Honolulu, USA (2015)
13. Bohland, J.W., Bokil, H., Allen, C.B., Mitra, P.P.: The brain atlas concordance problem: quantitative comparison of anatomical parcellations. PLoS ONE 4, e7200 (2009)
14. Jones, S.E., Buchbinder, B.R., Aharon, I.: Three-dimensional mapping of cortical thickness using laplace's equation. Hum. Brain Mapping 11, 12–32 (2000)
15. Leprince, Y., Poupon, F., Delzescaux, T., Hasboun, D., Poupon, C., Riviere, D.: Combined laplacian-equivolumic model for studying cortical lamination with ultra high field MRI (7T). In: 12th IEEE International Symposium on Biomedical Imaging, pp. 580–583. IEEE Press, New York (2015)
16. Lowe, D.G.: Distinctive image features from scale-invariant keypoints. Int. J. Comput. Vis. 60, 91–110 (2004)
17. Toews, M., Wells, W.M.: Efficient and robust model-to-image alignment using 3D scale-invariant features. Med. Image Anal. 17, 271–282 (2013)
18. Scovanner, P., Ali, S., Shah, M.: A 3-dimensional SIFT descriptor and its application to action recognition. In: Proceedings of the 15th ACM International Conference on Multimedia, pp. 357–360. AMC Press, New York (2007)
19. Golias, N.A., Dutton, R.W.: Delaunay triangulation and 3D adaptive mesh generation. Finite Elements Anal. Des. 25, 331–341 (1997)
20. Cha, S.H.: Comprehensive survey on distance/similarity measures between probability density functions. Int. J. Math. Models Methods Appl. Sci. 1, 300–307 (2007)

21. Mahalanobis, P.C.: On the generalised distance in statistics. Proc. Natl. Inst. Sci. India **2**, 49–55 (1936)
22. Hawrylycz, M.J., Lein, E.S., Guillozet-Bongaarts, A.L., Shen, E.H., Ng, L., Miller, J.A., van de Lagemaat, L.N., Smith, K.A., Ebbert, A., Riley, Z.L., et al.: An anatomically comprehensive atlas of the adult human brain transcriptome. Nature **489**, 391–399 (2012)
23. Shannon, C.E.: A mathematical theory of communication. Bell Labs Tech. J. **27**, 379–423 (1948)

LATEST: Local AdapTivE and Sequential Training for Tissue Segmentation of Isointense Infant Brain MR Images

Li Wang[1], Yaozong Gao[1,2], Gang Li[1], Feng Shi[1], Weili Lin[3], and Dinggang Shen[1(✉)]

[1] IDEA Lab, Department of Radiology and BRIC,
University of North Carolina at Chapel Hill, Chapel Hill, NC, USA
dinggang_shen@med.unc.edu
[2] Department of Computer Science, University of North Carolina at Chapel Hill,
Chapel Hill, NC, USA
[3] MRI Lab, Department of Radiology and BRIC,
University of North Carolina at Chapel Hill, Chapel Hill, NC, USA

Abstract. Accurate segmentation of isointense infant (~ 6 months of age) brain MRIs is of great importance, however, a very challenging task, due to extremely low tissue contrast caused by ongoing myelination processes. In this work, we propose a novel learning method based on Local AdapTivE and Sequential Training (LATEST) for segmentation. Specifically, random forest technique is employed to train a *local classifier* (a single decision tree) for each voxel in the common space based on the neighboring training samples from atlases. *Then*, for each given voxel, all trained nearby individual classifiers (decision trees) are grouped together to form a forest. Moreover, the estimated probabilities are further used as additional source images to train the next set of local classifiers for refining tissue classification. By iteratively training the subsequent classifiers based on the updated tissue probability maps, *a sequence of local classifiers* can be built for accurate tissue segmentation.

1 Introduction

The first year of life is the most dynamic phase of the postnatal human brain development, with rapid tissue growth and development of a wide range of cognitive and motor functions. Accurate tissue segmentation of infant brain MR images into white matter (WM), gray matter (GM), and cerebrospinal fluid (CSF) in this phase is of great importance for studying both normal and abnormal early brain development [1]. However, the segmentation of infant brain MRI is very challenging, due to reduced tissue contrast [2], increased noise [3], severe partial volume effect [4], and the ongoing white matter myelination [2, 5]. Especially, due to the ongoing myelination, at around 6 months of age, which is often referred to as isointense phase [6], the infant brain image appears isointense and exhibits the extremely low tissue contrast in both T1- and T2-weighted MR images, thus posing significant challenges for automatic tissue segmentation.

© Springer International Publishing AG 2017
H. Müller et al. (Eds.): MCV/BAMBI 2016, LNCS 10081, pp. 26–34, 2017.
DOI: 10.1007/978-3-319-61188-4_3

Although many methods have been proposed for infant brain MR image segmentation, most of them focused on segmentation of neonatal brain images in the infantile phase (≤ 5 months) [2, 4, 5, 7, 8], where images have the relatively distinguishable contrast between WM and GM in T2-weighted MR images. In contrast, there are only few works [9–11] focusing on segmentation of isointense (at ~ 6 months of age) infant brain images. In recent work [9], the convolutional neural networks (CNN) method [9] was proposed to segment the isointense infant brain images; however, it can only be applied to 2D image slices, instead of 3D data. In the work of [10], a learning-based method was proposed to integrate information from both multi-modality images and the tentatively-estimated tissue probability maps for infant brain image segmentation. Specifically, random forest [12] was first used to train a multi-class tissue classifier based on the training subjects with multiple imaging modalities. This trained classifier provided initial tissue probability maps for each training subject. Inspired by the auto-context model [13, 14], the estimated tissue probability maps were further used as additional input images to train the next classifier, by combining the high-level multi-class context features (calculated from the estimated tissue probability maps) with the appearance features (calculated from multi-modality images) for refining tissue classification. By iteratively training the subsequent classifiers based on the updated tissue probability maps, a sequence of classifiers were obtained for tissue segmentation. However, the classifiers were trained globally, i.e., the training samples extracted from the entire atlases were mixed for training, and the same classifiers were applied for every voxel. As demonstrated in [15, 16], local spatially-adaptive classifiers can significantly improve the performance of global classifiers. However, only one-layer classifiers were trained in [15, 16]. Inspired by both of these works [10, 15, 16], we propose to train spatially-adaptive sequential classifiers for segmentation of isointense infant brain MR images, by taking advantage of both sequential [10] and spatially-adaptive [15, 16] training. Specifically, all the atlases are first registered into a common template space. Then, for each voxel in the common space, an individual tree is trained via random forest based on the spatially-neighboring training samples from the aligned atlases. Then, for each given voxel, all the nearby trained individual trees are grouped together to form a forest for estimating its tissue probabilities. The estimated probabilities are further used as additional source images to train the next-layer local classifiers, by combining the high-level multi-class context features (calculated from the previously estimated tissue probability maps) with the appearance features (calculated from multi-modality MR images) for refining tissue classification. Finally, these sequential and spatially-adaptive classifiers can be built for accurate tissue segmentation.

2   Method

2.1   Dataset and Image Preprocessing

T1- and T2-weighted MR images of 20 infants were acquired on a Siemens head-only 3T scanners with a circular polarised head coil. During the scan, infants were asleep, unsedated, and fitted with ear protection, with their heads secured in a vacuum-fixation device. T1-weighted MR images were acquired with 160 sagittal slices using parameters: TR/TE = 2000/3 ms and resolution = $1 \times 1 \times 1$ mm^3. T2-weighted MR images were obtained with 160 sagittal slices using parameters: TR/TE = 4000/299 ms and resolution = $1 \times 1 \times 1$ mm^3. For image preprocessing, T2 images were linearly aligned onto their corresponding T1 images. Afterwards, standard image preprocessing steps were performed before tissue segmentation, including intensity inhomogeneity correction [17] and histogram matching.

Accurate manual segmentation is of great importance for training classifiers in the learning-based segmentation methods. Due to low contrast and huge number of voxels in brain images, manual segmentation is very difficult and time-consuming. Hence, to generate reliable manual segmentations for isointense infant subjects, we first obtained automatic segmentation results using a publicly available software iBEAT (http://www.nitrc.org/projects/ibeat/). Then, based on these obtained automatic segmentation results, manual editing was carefully performed by an experienced neuroradiologist to correct errors by using ITK-SNAP [18]. Manual editing of each subject took approximately 3 h. The intra-rater reliability (3 repeats) for WM, GM and CSF is 0.932, 0.931, and 0.960, respectively, in terms of Dice ratio. These 20 images with their edited tissue segmentation maps were used as multiple infant brain atlases.

2.2 Local AdapTivE and Sequential Training (LATEST)

In this paper, random forest [12] is adopted as a multi-class classifier to produce a tissue probability map for each tissue type (i.e., WM, GM, and CSF) by voxel-wise classification. As a supervised learning method, our method consists of training and testing stages. In the *training stage*, all the atlases are *first* linearly registered to a common template space. *Then*, an individual tree is independently trained at each voxel in the common space. Specifically, for a given voxel (i.e., a red point in Fig. 1(a)), all its nearby samples in a specified neighborhood (i.e., blue square) are used together as training samples. In the *testing stage*, to estimate tissue probability at a given voxel (i.e., a red point in Fig. 1(b)), all the neighboring trained individual trees (i.e., within red square) are grouped together to form a forest for classification. To deal with the challenges of low tissue contrast, inspired by [10], an auto-context model [13, 14] is further adopted to iteratively refine the tissue probability maps, by including context information calculated from the previously-estimated tissue probability maps. By iteratively training local trees with *random forest* and *auto-context model* on both the multi-modalities (T1 and T2) and the updated tissue probability maps, we can train a sequence of local classifiers for infant brain segmentation. All these training steps are detailed below.

- **Step 1: Registration to a common template space**. In the training stage, all the atlases are linearly registered to a common template space. Their corresponding tissue labels are also warped into the common space. In the testing stage, the target image is similarly registered to the same common space. Therefore, the rough correspondences between atlases and target image are established, based on which the trained sequential and spatially-adaptive classifiers can be mapped into the target image for testing.
- **Step 2: Extraction of appearance and context features**. For each voxel in the common space, all its nearby samples from each aligned atlas are randomly selected

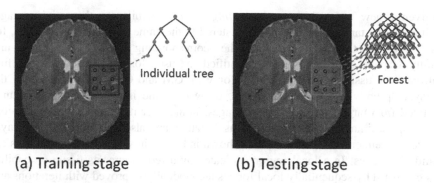

(a) Training stage   **(b) Testing stage**

Fig. 1. Illustration of training stage (a) and testing stage (b). In (a), the blue region denotes a neighborhood, within which all the voxels are used as training samples for the center red point. In (b), the red region denotes a neighborhood, where all trained individual trees are grouped together to form a forest in the testing stage. Note that the blue and red regions in (a) and (b) can have different sizes. (Color figure online)

as training samples. Then, we extract various features from each selected training sample for training the classifiers. Specifically, we extract appearance features from multi-modality MR images. Based on these extracted appearance features, we train the first-layer local classifier (with a single decision tree) for each voxel. Then, all the neighboring trained individual local classifiers are grouped together to form a forest for classification of each training sample, thus providing the initial tissue probability maps for each training atlas. Inspired by the auto-context model [14], we further extract context features from these initial tissue probability maps. Note that these context features are used to coordinate segmentations across different parts of multi-modality images, which have been shown effective in both computer vision and medical image analysis fields [19–22].

- **Step 3: Training of random-forest based local classifiers.** We train a local classifier to learn the complex relationship between local appearance/context features and the corresponding (manual ground-truth) tissue label on each selected training sample. Although many advanced classifiers have been developed, herein we adopt random forest [12] because of (1) its effectiveness in handling a large number of training data with high dimensionality and also (2) its fast speed in testing. Besides, random forest also allows us to explore a large number of image features to select the most suitable ones for accurate classification [23].
- **Step 4: Repeating Steps 2 and 3 until convergence.** Note that we train our local classifiers in a serial manner. Specifically, based on the local classifier trained in **Step 3**, all the neighboring individual trees are grouped together to form a forest for classification of each training voxel. By visiting each training voxel, we can update the tissue probability maps for each training atlas. Then, according to **Step 2**, we extract context features from the updated tissue probability maps, and further employ them along with the appearance features to train the next-layer local classifier for each voxel in the common space. Eventually, we will train and obtain sequential and spatially-adaptive classifiers for infant brain segmentation.

Given a new target image, *the testing stage* is similar to the training stage. Specifically, the target image is *first* registered to the same common space. *Then*, for each voxel in the target image, the corresponding trained sequential and spatially-adaptive classifiers will be identified and used for classification. In the first iteration, three tissue probability maps (for WM, GM and CSF) are estimated by the first-layer spatially-adaptive local forest, using only the image appearance features calculated from target multi-modality images. In the later iterations, the tissue probability maps estimated from the previous iteration are also fed into the next-layer classifier for refinement. An example is shown in Fig. 3, in which the input images are T1 and T2 images. In a local region indicated by a red square, its tissue probability maps estimated by sequentially local forests are gradually improved with iterations and become more and more accurate. It is worth noting that the result of first iteration can be regarded as the result obtained using only local classifiers in [15].

3   Experimental Results

We have evaluated the proposed method on 20 isointense infant subjects using leave-one-out cross-validation. The manual segmentation for each subject is considered as the "ground truth" for quantitative comparison. In our implementation, we use 3D random Haar-like features to compute both image appearance features and multi-class context features. Also, for each voxel, its neighborhood is defined as a 3D cube with size of $15 \times 15 \times 15$ for training, and $5 \times 5 \times 5$ for testing. For each tissue type, we select 2,000 training samples from the neighborhood for each training atlas. Then, for each training sample with the patch size of $7 \times 7 \times 7$, 10,000 random Haar-like features are extracted from all source images, i.e., T1- and T2-weighted MR images and also three probability maps of WM, GM, and CSF. As mentioned, for each voxel in the common space, we train one individual decision tree with conservative parameters setting, such as we stop the tree growth with maximal depth 50, or with a minimum of 8 sample numbers in each leaf node. We set the maximal iteration as 3 since we find the performance typically increases dramatically in the first 3 iterations, and then gradually after 3 iterations. In the following, we compare mainly with [10], since it achieves the state-of-the-art segmentation results on the 6-month infant brain MRIs.

Figure 3 shows the estimated probability maps by the proposed sequentially local classifiers in 3 iterations (#1–#3). As mentioned before, the classifiers in the first iteration of the proposed method can be considered as the local (one-step) classifiers (namely random forest based label fusion, *RFLF*) proposed in [15], and the corresponding results are shown in the third column (#1). Due to the absence of sequential training based on the intermediate tissue probabilities, the results by local (one-step) classifiers are noisy. The last column shows the result by sequential (global) classifiers (namely *LINKS*) proposed in [10]. Although the result by *LINKS* is free of noise, it is not accurate due to missing of local details. By contrast, the result by our proposed sequentially local classifiers is more accurate via visual observation, compared with the results by both local (one-step) classifiers [15] and sequential (global) classifiers [10].

Figure 2 shows the Dice ratios of WM, GM and CSF by sequentially applying the learned classifiers. It can be seen that the Dice ratios are improved with the iterations

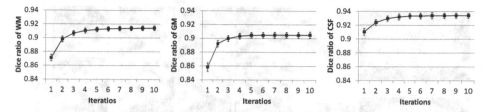

Fig. 2. Changes of Dice ratios of WM, GM and CSF with respect to the iteration number.

and become stable after a few iterations (i.e., 5 iterations), as reflected by the reduced standard deviation. These results demonstrate the importance of using iterative training.

In the following, we will make comparisons with (a) local (one-step) classifiers [15], (b) sequential (global) classifiers [10], and (c) manual segmentations. Figure 4 shows the segmentation results for a typical isointense infant subject by different methods. The first row shows the original T1 and T2 MRIs with manual segmentation. The second, third and fourth rows show the segmentation results by local (one-step) classifiers [15], sequential (global) classifiers [10], and our proposed sequentially local classifiers, respectively. For a fair comparison, we have trained sequential (global) classifiers [10] with optimised parameters on the warped atlases. As we can see, the result by the proposed method is more accurate than all other methods, particularly for the places indicated by dashed circles. Last two columns of Fig. 4 also show the segmented WM/GM rendering results (along with zoomed views) by different methods. As we can see, our result is more consistent with manual segmentations. Then, we further employ Dice ratios to evaluate the performances of different methods on 20 subjects, as given in Table 1. Besides Dice ratio, we also measured the modified Hausdorff distance (MHD), which is defined as the 95th percentile Hausdorff distance. It can be clearly seen that our proposed method outperforms all other methods.

4   Discussion and Conclusion

We have presented a novel learning method based on local adaptive and sequential training (LATEST) for tissue segmentation of isointense infant brain MR images. The key idea is to train spatially-adaptive and sequential classifiers. Specifically, a first-layer local classifier was first trained for each voxel in the common space. The classification results from neighboring classifiers are average to generate intermediate tissue probability maps, which were further used as additional source images to train the next-layer classifier. By iteratively training the subsequent classifiers based on the updated tissue probability maps, a sequence of local classifiers were built for accurate tissue segmentation. Experimental results on 20 isointense infant subjects show that the proposed method achieves better performance than the state-of-the-art methods.

It is worth noting that the neighborhood size is important for training. In our experiments, we found the performance dropped when using larger size of neighborhood. This is mainly because the use of larger neighborhood complicates the classification

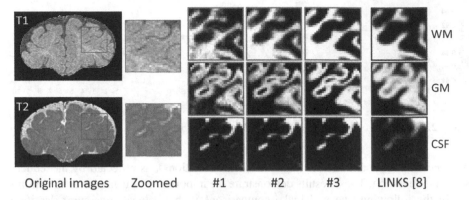

Fig. 3. The estimated probability maps by the proposed sequentially local forests along the iterations (#1–#3). #1 can also be considered as the result by using only local classifiers [15]. The last column shows the result by *LINKS* which uses sequentially global classifiers [10].

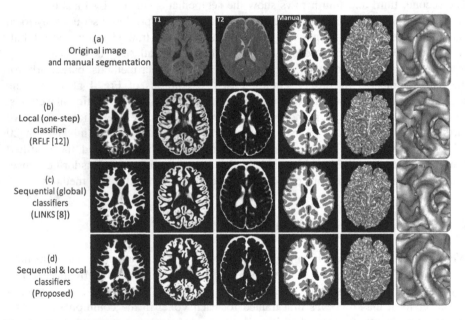

Fig. 4. Comparison of segmentation results on (a) a typical subject by (b) local (one-step) classifiers (*RFLF* [15]), (c) sequential (global) classifiers (*LINKS* [10]), and (d) our sequential & local classifiers (Proposed). The first row shows the T1 and T2 MR images and also manual segmentation. From left to right, the figure shows estimated the probabilities of WM, GM, and CSF, entire brain segmentation, 3D rendering, and zoomed 3D rendering, by three methods.

problem by including more irrelevant samples into training set. This observation also shows the importance of training local classifiers for accurate segmentation.

There are still some limitations for the proposed work. First, the proposed work cannot guarantee a correct topology result. Thus the post processing such as topology correction may be needed. Second, during the training, more samples should be selected from these incorrectly labeled voxels. Third, the Haar-like features are selected from one scale (patch size), which is not optimal since different structures have different scales.

Table 1. Average Dice ratios (in percentage) and MHD by 3 different methods on 20 isointense infant images. The bold indicates that the results by the proposed method are significantly better than others (p-value < 0.001).

Method		*RFLF* [15]: local (one-step)	*LINKS* [10]: sequential (global)	*Proposed*: sequential & local
Dice ratio	WM	84.6 ± 0.76	88.7 ± 0.43	**91.4 ± 0.33**
	GM	85.9 ± 0.88	87.1 ± 0.66	**90.5 ± 0.45**
	CSF	88.2 ± 0.41	89.3 ± 0.34	**93.4 ± 0.36**
MHD	WM/GM	2.57 ± 0.69	1.59 ± 0.25	**1.24 ± 0.28**
	GM/CSF	3.81 ± 0.78	1.89 ± 0.33	**1.50 ± 0.21**

Acknowledgements. This work was supported in part by National Institutes of Health grants (MH100217, MH070890, EB006733, EB008374, EB009634, AG041721, AG042599, MH088520, MH108914, MH107815, and MH109773).

References

1. Isgum, I., Benders, M.I.N.I., Avants, B., Cardoso, M.J., Counsell, S.J., Gomez, E.F., Gui, L., Huppi, P.S., Kersbergen, K.J., Makropoulos, A., Melbourne, A., Moeskops, P., Mol, C. P., Kuklisova-Murgasova, M., Rueckert, D., Schnabel, J.A., Srhoj-Egekher, V., Wu, J., Wang, S., de Vries, L.S., Viergever, M.A.: Evaluation of automatic neonatal brain segmentation algorithms: the NeoBrainS12 challenge. Med. Image Anal. **20**, 135–151 (2015)
2. Weisenfeld, N.I., Warfield, S.K.: Automatic segmentation of newborn brain MRI. NeuroImage **47**, 564–572 (2009)
3. Ruf, A., Greenspan, H., Goldberger, J.: Tissue classification of noisy MR brain images using constrained GMM. In: Duncan, J.S., Gerig, G. (eds.) MICCAI 2005. LNCS, vol. 3750, pp. 790–797. Springer, Heidelberg (2005). doi:10.1007/11566489_97
4. Xue, H., Srinivasan, L., Jiang, S., Rutherford, M., Edwards, A.D., Rueckert, D., Hajnal, J.V.: Automatic segmentation and reconstruction of the cortex from neonatal MRI. NeuroImage **38**, 461–477 (2007)
5. Gui, L., Lisowski, R., Faundez, T., Hüppi, P.S., Lazeyras, F.O., Kocher, M.: Morphology-driven automatic segmentation of MR images of the neonatal brain. Med. Image Anal. **16**, 1565–1579 (2012)
6. Paus, T., Collins, D.L., Evans, A.C., Leonard, G., Pike, B., Zijdenbos, A.: Maturation of white matter in the human brain: a review of magnetic resonance studies. Brain Res. Bull. **54**, 255–266 (2001)
7. Wang, L., Shi, F., Li, G., Gao, Y., Lin, W., Gilmore, J.H., Shen, D.: Segmentation of neonatal brain MR images using patch-driven level sets. Neuroimage **84**, 141–158 (2014)
8. Wang, L., Shi, F., Lin, W., Gilmore, J.H., Shen, D.: Automatic segmentation of neonatal images using convex optimization and coupled level sets. Neuroimage **58**, 805–817 (2011)

9. Zhang, W.L., Li, R.J., Deng, H.T., Wang, L., Lin, W.L., Ji, S.W., Shen, D.G.: Deep convolutional neural networks for multi-modality isointense infant brain image segmentation. Neuroimage **108**, 214–224 (2015)
10. Wang, L., Gao, Y., Shi, F., Li, G., Gilmore, J.H., Lin, W., Shen, D.: LINKS: learning-based multi-source IntegratioN frameworK for segmentation of infant brain images. Neuroimage **108**, 160–172 (2015)
11. Wang, L., Shi, F., Gao, Y., Li, G., Gilmore, J.H., Lin, W., Shen, D.: Integration of sparse multi-modality representation and anatomical constraint for isointense infant brain MR image segmentation. Neuroimage **89**, 152–164 (2014)
12. Breiman, L.: Random forests. Mach. Learn. **45**, 5–32 (2001)
13. Tu, Z., Bai, X.: Auto-context and its application to high-level vision tasks and 3D brain image segmentation. PAMI **32**, 1744–1757 (2010)
14. Loog, M., Ginneken, B.: Segmentation of the posterior ribs in chest radiographs using iterated contextual pixel classification. IEEE Trans. Med. Imaging **25**, 602–611 (2006)
15. Wang, H., Cao, Yu., Syeda-Mahmood, T.: Multi-atlas segmentation with learning-based label fusion. In: Wu, G., Zhang, D., Zhou, L. (eds.) MLMI 2014. LNCS, vol. 8679, pp. 256–263. Springer, Cham (2014). doi:10.1007/978-3-319-10581-9_32
16. Bai, W., Shi, W., Ledig, C., Rueckert, D.: Multi-atlas segmentation with augmented features for cardiac MR images. Med. Image Anal. **19**, 98–109 (2015)
17. Sled, J.G., Zijdenbos, A.P., Evans, A.C.: A nonparametric method for automatic correction of intensity nonuniformity in MRI data. IEEE Trans. Med. Imaging **17**, 87–97 (1998)
18. Yushkevich, P.A., Piven, J., Hazlett, H.C., Smith, R.G., Ho, S., Gee, J.C., Gerig, G.: User-guided 3D active contour segmentation of anatomical structures: Significantly improved efficiency and reliability. NeuroImage **31**, 1116–1128 (2006)
19. Sutton, C., McCallum, A., Rohanimanesh, K.: Dynamic conditional random fields: Factorized probabilistic models for labeling and segmenting sequence data. J. Mach. Learn. Res. **8**, 693–723 (2007)
20. Oliva, A., Torralba, A.: The role of context in object recognition. Trends Cogn. Sci. **11**, 520–527 (2007)
21. Belongie, S., Malik, J., Puzicha, J.: Shape matching and object recognition using shape contexts. IEEE Trans. Pattern Anal. Mach. Intell. **24**, 509–522 (2002)
22. Geman, S., Geman, D.: Stochastic relaxation, Gibbs distributions, and the Bayesian restoration of images. IEEE Trans. Pattern Anal. Mach. Intell. **6**, 721–741 (1984)
23. Zikic, D., Glocker, B., Criminisi, A.: Encoding atlases by randomized classification forests for efficient multi-atlas label propagation. Med. Image Anal. **18**, 1262–1273 (2014)

Landmark-Based Alzheimer's Disease Diagnosis Using Longitudinal Structural MR Images

Jun Zhang[1], Mingxia Liu[1], Le An[1], Yaozong Gao[1,2], and Dinggang Shen[1,3(✉)]

[1] Department of Radiology and BRIC, UNC at Chapel Hill, Chapel Hill, NC, USA
dgshen@med.unc.edu
[2] Department of Computer Science, UNC at Chapel Hill, Chapel Hill, NC, USA
[3] Department of Brain and Cognitive Engineering,
Korea University, Seoul, Republic of Korea

Abstract. In this paper, we propose a landmark-based feature extraction method for AD diagnosis using longitudinal structural MR images, which requires no nonlinear registration or tissue segmentation in the application stage and is robust to the inconsistency among longitudinal scans. Specifically, (1) the discriminative landmarks are first automatically discovered from the whole brain, which can be efficiently localized using a fast landmark detection method for the testing images; (2) High-level statistical spatial features and contextual longitudinal features are then extracted based on those detected landmarks. Using the spatial and longitudinal features, a linear support vector machine (SVM) is adopted for distinguishing AD subjects from healthy controls (HCs) and also mild cognitive impairment (MCI) subjects from HCs, respectively. Experimental results demonstrate the competitive classification accuracies, as well as a promising computational efficiency.

1 Introduction

Structural MRI has been proven to be an effective tool for Alzheimer's disease (AD) diagnosis [1]. Compared with cross-sectional study at a single time point, longitudinal study is more sensitive to early pathological changes by focusing on both the spatial structural abnormalities and the longitudinal variations of tissues.

So far, researches that focus on cross-sectional study have obtained several achievements on AD or mild cognitive impairment (MCI) diagnosis [2,3]. For example, Liu *et al.* investigated the AD diagnosis using multi-template representation [4–6]. Hinrichs *et al.* proposed to use spatially augmented LPboosting for AD classification [7]. Zhu *et al.* focused on selecting informative features from redundant region-based features [8–10]. Gerardin *et al.* extracted features based on hippocampal shape for the purpose of classifying AD and MCI [11]. Gao *et al.* proposed to use hypergraph learning for MCI classification and indexing [12,13]. Kloppe *et al.* proposed to use voxel-based gray matter features for AD classification [14].

On the other hand, existing longitudinal studies largely focus on the degeneration of well-known representative biomarkers including hippocampal volume,

© Springer International Publishing AG 2017
H. Müller et al. (Eds.): MCV/BAMBI 2016, LNCS 10081, pp. 35–45, 2017.
DOI: 10.1007/978-3-319-61188-4_4

ventricular volume, whole brain volume and cortical thickness. For example, Chincarini *et al.* proposed four image analysis strategies based on hippocampal volume by integrating longitudinal atrophy rate as a measurement for AD diagnosis [15]. Jack *et al.* investigated the changing rates of four structures (*i.e.*, hippocampus, entorhinal cortex, whole brain and ventricle), and supported the idea of using changing rates as biomarkers for AD diagnosis [16]. Aguilar *et al.* analyzed the longitudinal atrophy changes in cortical thickness measures and subcortical volumes, and pointed out that the use of two time points data yielded better index result compared with using the cross-sectional data only [17]. Kim *et al.* adopted 93 ROI features for longitudinal analysis [18]. However, there are still several challenges in existing longitudinal analysis: (1) Limited measurements may be incapable of capturing the full pattern of morphological abnormalities from the whole brain; (2) Time-consuming nonlinear registration or tissue segmentation step is required, and the longitudinal study exacerbates the computational time since more scans are involved; (3) Longitudinal scans across subjects are usually inconsistent, since some time points might be missing during the data collection.

In this study, a landmark-based feature extraction framework is proposed for AD diagnosis using longitudinal structural MR images. Different from traditional longitudinal studies, our method (1) does not require the time-consuming nonlinear registration or tissue segmentation, (2) can cover the representative morphological abnormalities from the whole brain, and (3) is able to handle the inconsistency among longitudinal scans. Specifically, the discriminative landmarks which have significant morphological group differences are automatically discovered from the whole brain. By using a regression forest-based landmark detection method, these landmarks can be efficiently detected in the application stage. Based on these detected landmarks, high-level spatial features and contextual longitudinal features are further extracted respectively, as below. (a) A bag-of-words strategy is used to extract high-level spatial features, by calculating the frequency of low-level landmark-based morphological features from different scanning time points. In this way, the significant spatial abnormalities from all scanning time points are aggregated together, which are also invariant to the number of longitudinal scans. (b) To extract contextual longitudinal features, an interpolation step is used to generate a Jacobian map from longitudinal landmark displacements. Then, contextual features can be extracted around the landmarks from the Jacobian map. Finally, a linear support vector machine (SVM) is adopted to perform AD/MCI classification using these spatial and longitudinal features.

2   Materials and Image Processing

2.1   Dataset

The Alzheimer's Disease Neuroimaging Initiative (ADNI)[1] is a 5-year public-private partnership to test whether serial MRI, positron emission tomography

---

[1] www.adni-info.org.

Table 1. Demographic information of selected subjects in the ADNI database

	Male/Female	Age (years) (Mean ± SD)	Edu. (years) (Mean ± SD)
AD	81/73	75.10 ± 7.50	14.82 ± 3.08
MCI	219/127	74.33 ± 9.91	15.53 ± 3.29
HC	111/96	75.83 ± 4.98	16.10 ± 2.86

Table 2. Number of scans for the selected subjects in the ADNI database

	3 scans	4 scans	5 scans	6 scans
AD	63	91	-	-
MCI	57	97	170	22
HC	46	145	16	-

(PET), other biological markers, and clinical and neuropsychological assessment can be combined to measure the progression of mild cognitive impairment and early Alzheimer's disease. One goal of ADNI is to develop improved methods that will lead to uniform standards for acquiring longitudinal, multi-site MRI and PET data on subjects with AD, MCI, and elderly healthy controls (HCs).

Subjects used in this study are from the ADNI-1 database. In this paper, we selected the subjects with at least three scanning time points of structural MRI, thus resulting in 207 age-matched HCs, 154 AD, and 346 MCI subjects. The demographic information (i.e., gender, age, and education) of the studied subjects used in this study are summarized in Table 1. The statistics of scans for the studied subjects is summarized in Table 2.

2.2   Image Processing

The image processing includes two major steps: linear alignment and landmark discovery.

Linear Alignment: All images are linearly aligned to a common template, namely Colin27, which was created by averaging 27 registered scans of a single subject [19]. In order to achieve high efficiency, we adopt a landmark-based affine registration method. Specifically, five pre-defined landmarks (i.e., anterior commissure (AC) and posterior commissure (PC) landmarks, and the other three representative landmarks in mid-sagittal plane) are automatically detected by a pre-trained regression forest-based landmark detection model. A global similarity transformation matrix, which encodes 7 degree of freedom (DOF), can be estimated between the landmarks from the moving image to the template. Since each landmark has 3 coordinate values, 5 landmarks are enough to estimate the transformation matrix.

Landmark Discovery: Our target is to identify the regions with group differences in local structures between patients and HCs. To this end, we intend to perform a voxel-wise group comparison between those two groups. However, the linearly aligned images are not voxel-wisely comparable. In order to build the correspondence among voxels from different images, all images are nonlinearly aligned to the Colin27 template after linear alignment. In general, the warped images are very similar to each other so that the subject-specific structural information in different images may not be significant. Therefore, we extract patch-based morphological features (*i.e.*, 3D histogram of orientation (HOG) features [20]) from the linearly aligned images to describe the local structures. By using the deformation field from nonlinear registration, we can build the correspondence between voxels in the template and all linearly aligned images. Therefore, for each voxel in the template, we can extract two groups of HOG features from its corresponding voxels in all training patients and HCs, respectively. We then perform the multivariate test, namely Hotelling's T^2 statistic [21], on the two groups, through which a p-value can be calculated for each voxel in the template. Accordingly, a p-value map can be obtained according to the template. Finally, the local minima from the p-value map are identified as locations of discriminative landmarks in the template space. More details on landmark discovery can be found in our previous work [22].

Then, these landmarks, which are located in the template space, can be directly projected to all training images using their deformation fields. For testing images, in order to avoid the time-consuming nonlinear registration, we train a regression forest-based landmark detector [23,24] to detect these landmarks. In this way, both training images and testing images would have same landmarks, and particularly, the landmarks for the testing images can be obtained efficiently, thanks to the fast landmark detector.

3   Feature Extraction

Based on the identified landmarks, we propose a landmark-based framework for extracting features from longitudinal MR images. Specifically, two types of landmark-based features, *i.e.*, spatial features and longitudinal features, are extracted to describe the spatial structural abnormalities and longitudinal landmark variations, respectively. In the following, we explain the details about the extraction process for each feature type.

3.1   Landmark-Based Spatial Feature Extraction

Intuitively, in cross-sectional study, the morphological features (*e.g.*, 3D HOG) for all landmarks can be extracted and concatenated as strong features for classification. However, there are two challenges in longitudinal study: (1) The numbers of scanning time points across subjects are inconsistent due to missing time points, and thus, it is difficult to extract a unified feature representation from different number of scans. (2) It is difficult to identify the corresponding baseline images across subjects, which means a baseline scanning time point of one subject may not correspond to that of another subject. How to extract a unified

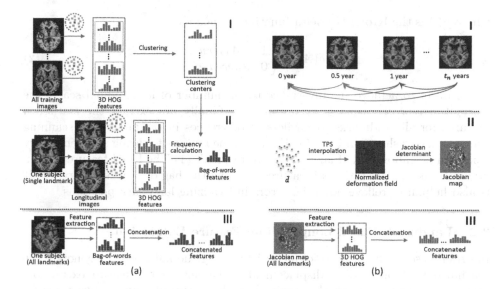

Fig. 1. Landmark-based feature extraction steps. (a) Spatial features. (b) Longitudinal features.

spatial feature representation from those inconsistent longitudinal scans is a very challenging task.

To address these two problems, we propose to use a bag-of-words strategy to extract statistical high-level spatial features. The bag-of-words strategy has demonstrated impressive performance on text, language, and image classification [25–28]. Specifically, Fig. 1(a) shows the procedure of our spatial feature extraction method, where each landmark is treated independently. As shown in Fig. 1(a) I, we first extract the 3D HOG feature vector for each landmark, as well as 3D HOG feature vectors for the supplementary voxels (*i.e.*, the neighboring voxels within a small spherical patch of the landmark). After extracting features from all training images and aggregating them together, we have a set of 3D HOG feature vectors. Then, we perform K-means clustering [29] on this set of feature vectors, and build a dictionary (*i.e.*, $\mathcal{D}$) with its *words* (*i.e.*, $\mathbf{w}_1, \mathbf{w}_2, \ldots, \mathbf{w}_M$) being the clustering centers. Then, for each individual subject, we can first extract the 3D HOG feature vectors (denoted by a feature set $\mathcal{F}$) for each landmark and its supplementary voxels in all longitudinal scans. The statistical histogram representation is then calculated by counting the occurrence frequencies of the clustering centers in these HOG features (*i.e.*, $\mathcal{F}$), as shown in Fig. 1(a) II. Mathematically, the histogram representation (*i.e.*, R) for one landmark can be defined as

$$R(j) = \sum_{\mathbf{f} \in \mathcal{F}} \delta((\operatorname*{argmin}_{i \in \{1,\ldots,M\}} \|\mathbf{f} - \mathbf{w}_i\|_2^2) = j), \ j = 1, \ldots, M, \tag{1}$$

where $\delta(\cdot)$ is the Kronecker delta function defined as

$$\delta(A) = \begin{cases} 1 \ if \ A \ is \ true; \\ 0 \ otherwise. \end{cases} \tag{2}$$

In order to achieve the invariance to the number of longitudinal scans, the histogram representation is ℓ_1 normalized. Finally, we extract the statistical features for all landmarks, regardless of differences in the number of scanning time points, as shown in Fig. 1(a) III. Here, the reasons for using supplementary voxels in neighborhood of landmarks are two-fold: (1) The HOG feature set can be expanded to get statistical features by using the bag-of-word strategy; (2) It is also helpful to relieve potential errors in localizing landmark positions.

3.2   Landmark-Based Longitudinal Feature Extraction

In order to solve the problem of inconsistent longitudinal scans, we generate the normalized 3D longitudinal displacement at the beginning of feature extraction. Specifically, we first define the longitudinal displacement between two scans for one specific landmark as follows:

$$d_{i,j} = L_{t_i} - L_{t_j}, \tag{3}$$

where L_{t_i} is the landmark location of the i-th scan from all longitudinal scans and t_i is the corresponding relative scanning time point with respect to the first scan. Then, the normalized 3D displacement $\bar{d}$ (mean displacement per year) is calculated from all possible combinations between two scans in different scanning time points, as shown in Fig. 1(b) I. Mathematically, $\bar{d}$ is defined as follows:

$$\bar{d} = \frac{1}{\sum_{1 \leq j < i \leq n} 1} \sum_{1 \leq j < i \leq n} \frac{d_{i,j}}{t_i - t_j}, \tag{4}$$

where n is the number of existing scans. As shown in Fig. 1(b) II, a normalized deformation field can be built by applying thin plate splines (TPS) interpolation to the normalized 3D longitudinal displacement $\bar{d}$ of all landmarks. Based on this normalized deformation field, a Jacobian map is further calculated to describe the longitudinal volume variations. Finally, as shown in Fig. 1(b) III, we can extract morphological features (*i.e.*, 3D HOG) for the landmarks in the Jacobian map. Therefore, longitudinal volume variations on these discriminative landmarks can be captured by these morphological features. It is worth noting that, instead of treating each landmark individually, the neighboring landmarks are jointed together with interpolation during the generation of the normalized deformation field. In this way, although the morphological features from Jacobian map are extracted for each landmark individually, the contextual information about the neighboring landmarks is automatically embedded into the calculated features.

4   Experiments

4.1   Parameter Setup

Using a 10-fold cross validation strategy, we conducted experiments for two classification tasks, *i.e.*, AD vs. HC and MCI vs. HC. The parameters in our approach were defined as follows: For 3D HOG feature extraction, we used 9 orientations, $2 \times 2 \times 2$ cells, and a size of $8 \times 8 \times 8$ for each cell. Therefore, the dimensionality of 3D HOG features was 72. In the bag-of-words strategy, the number of clustering centers was set to 50, and thus, the dimensionality of spatial features for each landmark was 50. The radius of spherical patch for sampling supplementary voxels was 5. For SVM classification, we fixed the margin parameter $C = 1$. Due to the data-driven property of our method, the number of landmarks was determined by the training images. In our method, we searched the local minima within a $7 \times 7 \times 7$ cubic patch, and obtained roughly 1500 identified landmarks for each fold in the cross validation.

4.2   Experimental Results

Five classification performance measures were used, namely (1) accuracy (ACC): the number of correctly classified samples divided by the total number of samples; (2) sensitivity (SEN): the number of correctly classified positive samples (patients) divided by the total number of positive samples; (3) specificity (SPE): the number of correctly classified negative samples (controls) divided by the total number of negative samples; and (4) balanced accuracy (BAC): the mean value of sensitivity and specificity; (5) area under receiver operating characteristic (ROC) curve (AUC).

For comparison, we also report the classification results of two baseline strategies based on our landmarks. The baseline spatial features are the HOG features that are directly extracted according to the landmarks only from the baseline

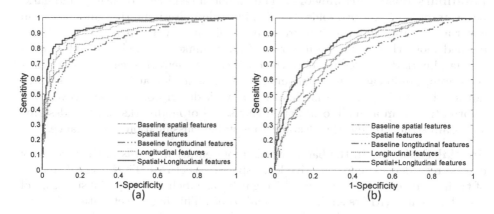

Fig. 2. ROC curves for classification. (a) AD vs. HC. (b) MCI vs. HC.

Table 3. Classification results achieved by methods using different features.

	AD vs. HC (%)					MCI vs. HC (%)				
	ACC	SEN	SPE	BAC	AUC	ACC	SEN	SPE	BAC	AUC
Baseline spatial features	84.40	74.34	91.79	83.06	91.98	74.86	84.68	58.45	71.5	80.78
Spatial features	86.35	77.63	92.75	85.19	92.52	76.49	86.13	**60.39**	73.26	84.57
Baseline longitudinal features	78.83	72.37	83.57	77.97	84.64	69.08	78.32	53.62	65.97	73.04
Longitudinal features	80.78	77.63	83.09	80.36	87.69	72.88	85.55	51.69	68.62	77.26
Spatial+Longitudinal features	**88.30**	**79.61**	**94.69**	**87.15**	**94.01**	**79.02**	**90.46**	59.90	**75.18**	**85.19**

MR image (first scan). The baseline longitudinal features refer to the features obtained by directly using normalized displacements (*i.e.*, $\bar{d}$) of the landmarks.

Table 3 reports the classification results, and Fig. 2 shows their corresponding ROC curves. These results demonstrate that, in both classification tasks, the proposed spatial features consistently outperform the baseline spatial features, and our longitudinal features generally achieve better performance than the baseline longitudinal features. Moreover, the combination of the proposed spatial and longitudinal features can further improve the classification performance.

In a related work, Chincarini et al. [15] used hippocampal volume and hippocampal volume atrophy rate as measurements for longitudinal AD classification. The reported AUC for AD vs. HC on ADNI-1 is 93.00%, which is slightly lower than ours (94.01%). Moreover, they used multi-atlas based method to obtain the hippocampal segmentations which is time-consuming. As we know, it usually takes hours to get accurate hippocampal segmentation. For our landmark-based method (*e.g.*, using four longitudinal scans), it takes less than 3 min to complete all feature extraction steps, including linear registration, landmark detection, and spatial and longitudinal feature extraction.

5   Discussions and Conclusions

Landmark-based Framework: The major advantages of using landmark-based framework are two folds: (1) The identified discriminative landmarks can cover all possible abnormalities from the whole brain without using several predefined biomarkers; (2) The use of landmarks makes it possible to integrate a fast landmark detection model to the diagnosis framework such that both time-consuming nonlinear registration and tissue segmentation are avoided. It is worth noting that, although each landmark is a weak descriptor that only covers the information from a small local patch, thousands of landmarks can well describe the brain structure and thus leading to a stable classification performance.

Spatial Features: In the bag-of-words representation, *words* in the dictionary can be regarded as representative local spatial structures. Thus, the calculation of their occurrence frequency can be regarded as labeling the spatial structure of each landmark with its similarities to all *words*. This high-level statistic ignores both the numbers and the orders of scanning time points and only focuses on the spatial abnormalities, which is suitable for extracting unified spatial features from inconsistent longitudinal scans. As can be seen in Table 3 and Fig. 2, the method of using bag-of-words based spatial features achieves better classification performance, compared with that using baseline spatial features.

Longitudinal Features: Intuitively, one type of longitudinal information is the trajectory of landmarks along time. However, the coherence among neighboring landmarks is ignored if we just simply use the mean longitudinal displacements ($\bar{d}$) as features. In our method, we generate a normalized deformation field by interpolation, through which the contextual information can be employed by jointly using the neighboring landmarks. Moreover, it is also well known that the Jacobian determinant can indicate the volume variation. Therefore, the morphological features from the Jacobian map comprehensively capture the longitudinal volume variation around landmarks. The experimental results show that using the longitudinal features from Jacobian map achieves 2% to 4% improvement in terms of accuracy as compared with the baseline longitudinal features.

Limitations and Future Work: Since each landmark has 72 spatial features and 50 longitudinal features, the concatenation of the features from all landmarks would be high dimensional, with respect to the number of training subjects. Also, there may be some redundant or noisy features that can adversely affect the classification model learning. Therefore, selecting most discriminative landmarks and features is important and will provide a reasonable solution for further performance improvement, which is our future work.

References

1. Frisoni, G.B., Fox, N.C., Jack, C.R., Scheltens, P., Thompson, P.M.: The clinical use of structural MRI in Alzheimer disease. Nat. Rev. Neurol. **6**(2), 67–77 (2010)
2. Thung, K.H., Wee, C.Y., Yap, P.T., Shen, D., Initiative, A.D.N., et al.: Neurodegenerative disease diagnosis using incomplete multi-modality data via matrix shrinkage and completion. NeuroImage **91**, 386–400 (2014)
3. Thung, K.-H., Yap, P.-T., Adeli-M, E., Shen, D.: Joint diagnosis and conversion time prediction of progressive mild cognitive impairment (PMCI) using low-rank subspace clustering and matrix completion. In: Navab, N., Hornegger, J., Wells, W.M., Frangi, A.F. (eds.) MICCAI 2015. LNCS, vol. 9351, pp. 527–534. Springer, Cham (2015). doi:10.1007/978-3-319-24574-4_63
4. Liu, M., Zhang, D., Shen, D.: View-centralized multi-atlas classification for Alzheimer's disease diagnosis. Hum. Brain Mapp. **36**(5), 1847–1865 (2015)
5. Liu, M., Zhang, D., Adeli-Mosabbeb, E., Shen, D.: Inherent structure based multiview learning with multi-template feature representation for Alzheimer's disease diagnosis. IEEE Trans. Biomed. Eng. **63**(7), 1473–1482 (2016)
6. Liu, M., Zhang, D., Shen, D.: Relationship induced multi-template learning for diagnosis of Alzheimer's disease and mild cognitive impairment. IEEE Trans. Med. Imaging **35**(6), 1463–1474 (2016)
7. Hinrichs, C., Singh, V., Mukherjee, L., Xu, G., Chung, M.K., Johnson, S.C., Initiative, A.D.N., et al.: Spatially augmented lpboosting for ad classification with evaluations on the adni dataset. Neuroimage **48**(1), 138–149 (2009)

8. Zhu, X., Suk, H.I., Shen, D.: A novel matrix-similarity based loss function for joint regression and classification in AD diagnosis. NeuroImage **100**, 91–105 (2014)
9. Zhu, X., Suk, H.I., Lee, S.W., Shen, D.: Canonical feature selection for joint regression and multi-class identification in Alzheimer's disease diagnosis. Brain Imaging Behav. **10**(3), 1–11 (2015)
10. Zhu, X., Suk, H.I., Lee, S.W., Shen, D.: Subspace regularized sparse multitask learning for multiclass neurodegenerative disease identification. IEEE Trans. Biomed. Eng. **63**(3), 607–618 (2016)
11. Gerardin, E., Chételat, G., Chupin, M., Cuingnet, R., Desgranges, B., Kim, H.S., Niethammer, M., Dubois, B., Lehéricy, S., Garnero, L., et al.: Multidimensional classification of hippocampal shape features discriminates alzheimer's disease and mild cognitive impairment from normal aging. Neuroimage **47**(4), 1476–1486 (2009)
12. Gao, Y., Adeli-M., E., Kim, M., Giannakopoulos, P., Haller, S., Shen, D.: Medical image retrieval using multi-graph learning for MCI diagnostic assistance. In: Navab, N., Hornegger, J., Wells, W.M., Frangi, A.F. (eds.) MICCAI 2015. LNCS, vol. 9350, pp. 86–93. Springer, Cham (2015). doi:10.1007/978-3-319-24571-3_11
13. Gao, Y., Wee, C.-Y., Kim, M., Giannakopoulos, P., Montandon, M.-L., Haller, S., Shen, D.: MCI identification by joint learning on multiple MRI data. In: Navab, N., Hornegger, J., Wells, W.M., Frangi, A.F. (eds.) MICCAI 2015. LNCS, vol. 9350, pp. 78–85. Springer, Cham (2015). doi:10.1007/978-3-319-24571-3_10
14. Klöppel, S., Stonnington, C.M., Chu, C., Draganski, B., Scahill, R.I., Rohrer, J.D., Fox, N.C., Jack, C.R., Ashburner, J., Frackowiak, R.S.: Automatic classification of MR scans in Alzheimer's disease. Brain **131**(3), 681–689 (2008)
15. Chincarini, A., Sensi, F., Rei, L., Gemme, G., Squarcia, S., Longo, R., Brun, F., Tangaro, S., Bellotti, R., Amoroso, N., et al.: Integrating longitudinal information in hippocampal volume measurements for the early detection of Alzheimer's disease. NeuroImage **125**, 834–847 (2016)
16. Jack, C., Shiung, M., Gunter, J., Obrien, P., Weigand, S., Knopman, D.S., Boeve, B.F., Ivnik, R.J., Smith, G.E., Cha, R., et al.: Comparison of different MRI brain atrophy rate measures with clinical disease progression in AD. Neurology **62**(4), 591–600 (2004)
17. Aguilar, C., Muehlboeck, J.S., Mecocci, P., Vellas, B., Tsolaki, M., Kloszewska, I., Soininen, H., Lovestone, S., Wahlund, L.O., Simmons, A., et al.: Application of a MRI based index to longitudinal atrophy change in Alzheimer disease, mild cognitive impairment and healthy older individuals in the addneuromed cohort. Front. Aging Neurosci. **6**, 145 (2014)
18. Thung, K.H., Wee, C.Y., Yap, P.T., Shen, D.: Identification of progressive mild cognitive impairment patients using incomplete longitudinal MRI scans. Brain Struct. Funct. 1–17 (2015)
19. Holmes, C.J., Hoge, R., Collins, L., Woods, R., Toga, A.W., Evans, A.C.: Enhancement of MR images using registration for signal averaging. J. Comput. Assist. Tomogr. **22**(2), 324–333 (1998)
20. Dalal, N., Triggs, B.: Histograms of oriented gradients for human detection. In: IEEE Computer Society Conference on Computer Vision and Pattern Recognition 2005. CVPR 2005, pp. 886–893. IEEE (2005)
21. Mardia, K.: Assessment of multinormality and the robustness of Hotelling's T^2 test. Appl. Stat. **24**, 163–171 (1975)
22. Zhang, J., Gao, Y., Gao, Y., Brent, M., Shen, D.: Detecting anatomical landmarks for fast Alzheimer's disease diagnosis. IEEE Trans. Med. Imaging **35**(12), 2524–2533 (2016)

23. Gao, Y., Shen, D.: Context-aware anatomical landmark detection: application to deformable model initialization in prostate CT images. In: Wu, G., Zhang, D., Zhou, L. (eds.) MLMI 2014. LNCS, vol. 8679, pp. 165–173. Springer, Cham (2014). doi:10.1007/978-3-319-10581-9_21

24. Zhang, J., Gao, Y., Wang, L., Tang, Z., Xia, J.J., Shen, D.: Automatic craniomaxillofacial landmark digitization via segmentation-guided partially-joint regression forest model and multi-scale statistical features. IEEE Trans. Biomed. Eng. **63**(9), 1820–1829 (2016)

25. Leung, T., Malik, J.: Representing and recognizing the visual appearance of materials using three-dimensional textons. Int. J. Comput. Vision **43**(1), 29–44 (2001)

26. Nowak, E., Jurie, F., Triggs, B.: Sampling strategies for bag-of-features image classification. In: Leonardis, A., Bischof, H., Pinz, A. (eds.) ECCV 2006. LNCS, vol. 3954, pp. 490–503. Springer, Heidelberg (2006). doi:10.1007/11744085_38

27. Yang, J., Jiang, Y.G., Hauptmann, A.G., Ngo, C.W.: Evaluating bag-of-visual-words representations in scene classification. In: Proceedings of the International Workshop on Multimedia Information Retrieval, pp. 197–206. ACM (2007)

28. Jiang, Y.G., Ngo, C.W., Yang, J.: Towards optimal bag-of-features for object categorization and semantic video retrieval. In: Proceedings of the 6th ACM International Conference on Image and Video Retrieval, ACM 494–501(2007)

29. Hartigan, J.A., Wong, M.A.: Algorithm AS 136: A k-means clustering algorithm. J. Roy. Stat. Soc.: Ser. C (Appl. Stat.) **28**(1), 100–108 (1979)

MCV Workshop: Lung Imaging

Inferring Disease Status by Non-parametric Probabilistic Embedding

Nematollah Kayhan Batmanghelich[1,2]([✉]), Ardavan Saeedi[1],
Raul San Jose Estepar[2], Michael Cho[2], and William M. Wells III[1,2]

[1] Computer Science and Artificial Intelligence Lab, MIT, Cambridge, USA
{kayhan,ardavans}@mit.edu
[2] Harvard Medical School, Brigham and Women's Hospital, Boston, USA
{rjosest,sw}@bwh.harvard.edu, remhc@channing.harvard.edu

Abstract. Computing similarity between all pairs of patients in a dataset enables us to group the subjects into disease subtypes and infer their disease status. However, robust and efficient computation of pairwise similarity is a challenging task for large-scale medical image datasets. We specifically target diseases where multiple subtypes of pathology present simultaneously, rendering the definition of the similarity a difficult task. To define pairwise patient similarity, we characterize each subject by a probability distribution that generates its local image descriptors. We adopt a notion of affinity between probability distributions which lends itself to similarity between subjects. Instead of approximating the distributions by a parametric family, we propose to compute the affinity measure indirectly using an approximate nearest neighbor estimator. Computing pairwise similarities enables us to embed the entire patient population into a lower dimensional manifold, mapping each subject from high-dimensional image space to an informative low-dimensional representation. We validate our method on a large-scale lung CT scan study and demonstrate the state-of-the-art prediction on an important physiologic measure of airflow (the forced expiratory volume in one second, FEV1) in addition to a 5-category clinical rating (so-called GOLD score).

1 Introduction

As the size of an image dataset grows, the chance of observing more phenotypically similar patients increases. This premise makes analysis of large-scale image datasets attractive: subject similarities can reveal subtypes or the underlying biology of disease. In addition to the computational challenges of large datasets, defining robust image similarity measures in the presence of significant anatomical variation is a difficult task. Our approach targets heterogeneous diseases where the pathology in each patient can be thought of as a superposition of different processes, or subtypes of a disease. We propose a method that is computationally efficient and statistically robust. Our motivation comes from a study of Chronic Obstructive Pulmonary Disease (COPD), but the resulting model is applicable to a wide range of heterogeneous disorders.

© Springer International Publishing AG 2017
H. Müller et al. (Eds.): MCV/BAMBI 2016, LNCS 10081, pp. 49–57, 2017.
DOI: 10.1007/978-3-319-61188-4_5

A common method to compute similarities is based on image registration. Gerber *et al.* [5] applied pairwise registrations and defined similarity based on geodesic distance on the Riemannian manifold of diffeomorphic transformations. Hamm *et al.* [6] proposed a similar method except they restricted their analysis to a smaller subset of transformations and incorporated the residual of the registration into the similarity measure. Both methods rely on pairwise registration which is computationally demanding in large-scale settings and less applicable in the presence of large variations in anatomy. Unlike brain abnormalities in Alzheimers disease, the lung abnormalities in COPD are scattered and less localized [10]. This renders the definition of similarity between two images more challenging.

One approach to this challenge is to model image content as a *set* of local features. More specifically in the context of lung disease, Sorensen *et al.* [16] use histogram and texture features of local patches to create a binary ab/normal classification and suggest aggregation of the posterior probabilities to a subject-level score. Similarly Toews *et al.* [17] propose to represent images as collections of scale-invariant features and construct an approximate nearest neighbor graph of local features. To infer the subject-level score, they sum the log-likelihood function of the class associated with observed image features. In both cases, the presence of the patch-level labels [16] or subject-level labels [17] is required to infer the patient score. It is not clear how those methods can be applied in an unsupervised fashion.

We propose a general method that aggregates similarities from local-level image descriptors to infer subject-level similarities. The local descriptors are viewed as samples from subject-specific probability distributions; therefore the similarity between subjects is naturally reduced to a notion of similarity between probability distributions which should be estimated from their observed samples. Although a parametric approach can be used to infer the distributions for each subject [1], estimating those parameters can be computationally expensive if only pairwise similarities are of interest. Also, a misspecified parametric family biases the similarity estimation. We adopt a non-parametric approach proposed by Wang *et al.* [19] where the computation of similarity only depends on distances of each local feature from its k-nearest neighbors and does not require kernel density estimators (KDE). Using fast methods to approximate a nearest neighbor graph [12] enables us to achieve computational efficiency comparable to that of Toews *et al.* [17]. Another advantage is that no patch- or subject-level labels are required hence the method can be applied in an unsupervised fashion (*e.g.*, for sub-typing).

We illustrate an application of the method on a large-scale study of COPD. Our method outperforms the state-of-the-art approach in predicting clinical values related to COPD. We show how this method is used to embed the patient population in a lower dimensional space and its effectiveness in capturing disease structure in the embedding space.

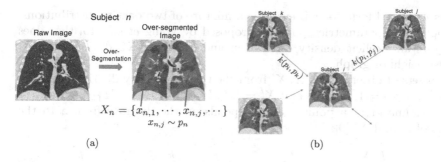

(a)   (b)

Fig. 1. (a) Feature extraction procedure for each subject. We extract local image descriptors (*e.g.*, $x_{n,j}$) from each super-pixel. X_n denotes the set of all local features from subject n. We model each subject with its corresponding probability density (*e.g.*, p_n). (b) Similarity graph between subjects. $k(p_i, p_j)$ denotes the similarity strength (affinity) between subjects i and j.

2   Method

In this section, we first describe the notation and the general setting. Then, we explain the algorithm to compute the pairwise patient similarities. Finally, we will explain how we use the similarity measurements to embed the patient population into a lower dimensional representation which is used to predict clinical values.

General Setting: Let each of $X_1, \cdots, X_N$ denote the *set* of local image features extracted from images of subjects $1, \cdots, N$ in the dataset. More specifically, we use an over-segmentation approach [7] to subdivide areas of a lung into groups of homogeneous super-pixels while preserving the boundaries of objects in the image. $X_n = \{x_{n,1}, \cdots, x_{n,m_n}\}$ is a set of image signatures extracted from m_n super-pixels where $x_{n,i} \in \mathbb{R}^d$ are local image descriptors extracted from region i of subject n. We will explore different options for the local descriptors in the experiment section of the paper. Following so-called "bag-of-words" representation [15], we model X_n as sample points from an unknown subject-specific distribution, $X_n \sim p_n$ (*i.e.*, $x_{n,i} \sim p_n$). We define similarity between subject i and subject j by defining a similarity measure between the corresponding distributions $k(p_i, p_j)$. We aim to estimate this quantity without estimating the underlying distribution. The general scheme is shown in Fig. 1.

Distance between Distributions: To define similarity between images of two subjects given their observed bags of local descriptors $X \sim p$, $X' \sim q$, we need to define similarity between their corresponding distributions. We first define the distance between distributions and convert it to a similarity measure. We use Kullback Leibler (KL) as the distance between distributions:

$$\mathrm{KL}(p\|q) = \int_{\mathbb{R}^d} \log \frac{p(x)}{q(x)} p(x) dx. \tag{1}$$

There is no closed-form for KL even for a mixture of two density distributions. We adopt a non-parametric approach proposed by Wang *et al.* [19] that does not require an explicit density estimation and estimates KL directly using a k-nearest neighbor graph.

Given sets of observations X, X' from the two probability distributions p, q, $X = \{x_i | x_i \sim p; i = 1, \cdots, N\}$ and $X' = \{x'_i | x'_i \sim q; i = 1, \cdots, M\}$, a k-nearest neighbor estimator of a point z only depends on the distance from z to the elements of X and X' [9]:

$$\hat{p}_k(z) = \frac{k/N}{\text{vol}(z, \rho_k(z))} = \frac{k}{Nc\rho_k^d(z)}, \quad \hat{q}_k(z) = \frac{k/M}{\text{vol}(z, \nu_k(z))} = \frac{k}{Mc\nu_k^d(z)}, \quad (2)$$

where $\text{vol}(x, R)$ is the volume of a ball of radius R centered at z, $\rho_k(z)$ and $\nu_k(z)$ are the distance from the k'th nearest neighbor of z in the sets X and X' respectively, and c stands for the volume of a d-dimensional unit ball.

An unbiased estimator for the $\text{KL}(p\|q)$ from the corresponding set of observed local descriptors, X and X' is the following:

$$\hat{\text{KL}}_{N,M}(p\|q) = \frac{d}{N} \sum_{n=1}^{N} \log \frac{\nu_k(x_n)}{\rho_k(x_n)} + \log \frac{M}{N-1}. \quad (3)$$

Notice that the method directly estimates KL without estimating p and q and it only depends on the k-nearest neighbor distances (*i.e.*, $\rho_k(\cdot)$, $\nu_k(\cdot)$). The approximate k-nearest neighbor graph is constructed efficiently using [12]. Wang *et al.* [19] proved the estimator is asymptotically unbiased: $\lim_{N,M \to \infty} \mathbb{E} \left[\hat{\text{KL}}_{N,M}(p\|q) \right] \to \text{KL}(p\|q)$.

Subject-level Score Vector and Prediction: Let matrix L denote exponentiated symmetric KL distance; *i.e.*, $L_{ij} = \exp\left(-\text{KL}_{\text{sym}}(X_i, X_j)/\sigma^2\right)$ where $\text{KL}_{\text{sym}}(X_i, X_j) = \hat{\text{KL}}(X_i \| X_j) + \hat{\text{KL}}(X_j \| X_i)$. $\hat{\text{KL}}(X_i \| X_j)$ is estimated using (3). We form the similarity kernel by projecting L on the positive definite cone as suggested by Chen *et al.* [4]. As suggested by Chang *et al.* [3], we set σ to the median value of the KL_{sym} in the dataset in all of our experiments.

Computing the similarity matrix enables us to employ an embedding method and project each subject to a lower dimensional space by unfolding the manifold space of the subjects. To do that, we apply the Cholesky decomposition on the similarity matrix and feed the resulting factorization to a Linear Embedding (LLE) [20] algorithm and derive a lower dimensional subject-specific score vector. The resulting vector will be used for prediction of clinical measurements and visualization.

3   Experiments

In this section, we apply our method to a large-scale study of a COPD. We validate our method by predicting clinical measurements related to COPD and characterizing the disease continuum. The goal of this experiment is to compare the proposed method with classical baselines and investigate its robustness with respect to different choices of local image descriptors.

We apply our method on various local image descriptors and compare our performance with a global baseline feature and a classical representation method. As a baseline feature, we use two clinically important CT measurements of lung density, INSP950 and EXP950. INSP950, the percentage of voxels < -950HU, is a quantitative measure of emphysema. EXP950, the percentage of voxels < -950HU after exhalation, reflects the degree of gas trapping [11, 14]. We also compare our approach with a classical representation method, Bag-of-Words (BoW), where images are represented by a histogram of words; words are clustered features from super-pixels. We used k-means clustering for BoW.

Data Preparation and Experimental Setting: We apply the method to CT images of lungs on 7292 subjects from the COPDGene study [13]. After automatic segmentation of the lung, we employ an over-segmentation approach [7] to subdivide areas of a lung into groups of spatially homogeneous super-pixels. We extract the following local features:

Histogram: Local histogram have been shown to be effective in characterizing emphysema [1, 2, 16]. We follow two procedures to extract histogram features. In the first, we extract a 32-bin histogram from each super-pixel (ref. as Hist32); 32 is roughly the third root of the average number of pixels in the super-pixel as suggested [16]. In the second procedure, we divide the histogram into 100 bins, followed by a PCA to reduce the dimensions to 30 (ref. as HistPCA) as suggested [1].

Texture: Texture features are shown to be important in characterizing lung tissue [16, 18]. Sorensen *et al.* [16] suggested using rotational invariant texture features. We adopt a rotation invariant histogram of gradient descriptors as proposed by Liu *et al.* [8]. Their method considers a gradient histogram as a continuous angular signal represented by the spherical harmonics (ref. as sHOG). We also extract Harilick features from the Gray-Level Co-occurrence Matrix (GLCM) following the pipeline [18] where the histogram information is already incorporated.

Evaluation: After computing the similarity matrix and the embedding vector scores (see Sect. 2), the resulting vectors are used as features in the following experiments. We use the Random Forest method to predict the GOLD score and linear Ridge regression (with the regularization weight set to 1) to estimate the continuous respiratory score (FEV1). Since neither of these clinical scores are derived from images, this experiment independently validates how well the embedding coordinates computed from the image similarity measure characterize the underlying disease process. We report r^2 and the Mean Squared Error (MSE) of the prediction of FEV1 and accuracy for GOLD score. We train on 99%, test on 1%, and repeat this process 50 times.

The results are reported in Table 1. All similarity-based predictions outperform the traditional threshold-based approach (*i.e.*, `Baseline`) irrespective of the local descriptors. To be comparable, we set the number of clusters in BoW to the dimensionality of our embedding method ($d = 100$). Our similarity-based representation outperforms BoW in r^2 and MSE and ties on accuracy. We computed p-values of the performance differences using a paired t-test. Our method is significantly better than the clinical image feature with $- \log p$-value$\gg$ 5. The $-\log p$-values of the difference between the best performances of BoW and our method for r^2, MSE, and accuracy are 3.4, 3.2, and 0.01 respectively. The significant performance difference between BoW and our method for `Harilick` descriptor demonstrates robustness of the method with respect to choice of texture feature.

Table 1. Mean and bootstrap 95% confidence interval width (in parentheses) of the prediction performance for `GOLD` score and `FEV1`. The best results are shown in bold. The six first rows are the baseline methods: global feature and the traditional Bag-of-Words representation respectively.

		FEV1		GOLD
	Image feature	r^2	MSE	% Accuracy
	Baseline	0.50 (0.03)	0.018 (0.001)	42.8 (1.5)
BoW	Hist32	0.51 (0.03)	0.018 (0.001)	47.2 (1.7)
	HistPCA	0.51 (0.04)	0.018 (0.001)	47.3 (1.5)
	Hist32+sHOG	0.56 (0.03)	0.016 (0.001)	47.2 (1.7)
	HistPCA+sHOG	0.51 (0.04)	0.018 (0.001)	**47.2 (1.3)**
	Harilick	0.33 (0.03)	0.025 (0.002)	39.6 (1.6)
Ours	Hist32	0.57 (0.03)	0.016 (0.001)	45.7 (1.5)
	HistPCA	0.57 (0.03)	0.015 (0.001)	47.1 (1.7)
	Hist32+sHOG	**0.59 (0.03)**	**0.015 (0.001)**	47.0 (1.8)
	HistPCA+sHOG	0.57 (0.03)	0.015 (0.001)	**47.3 (1.7)**
	Harilick	0.56 (0.03)	0.016 (0.001)	45.4 (1.6)

Figure 2 reports the effect of dimensionality of the representation on the prediction performance. Figure 2a shows the projection of patients on a 2D embedding space. A dot represents a patient and its color denotes `FEV1`. Even 2D embedding captures the structure of the disease; subjects on the bottom right are healthier than subjects on top left of the embedding space. Figure 2b reports the r^2 for `FEV1` with respect to dimensionality of the representation (*i.e.*, cluster size for BoW and embedding dim.) for `Hist32+sHOG` features. Both methods stabilize quickly in terms of performance and our method outperforms BoW.

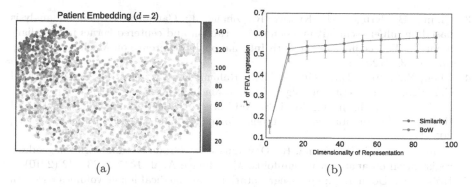

Fig. 2. (a) Embedding patients on a 2D space. A dot represents a patient and its color denotes FEV1 (severity of COPD). Hotter colors indicate more severe disease. (b) Prediction performance (r^2) of FEV1 with respect to the dimensionality of the embedding.

4 Conclusion

In this paper, we proposed to embed subject images into a manifold using an efficient pairwise similarity between probability distributions. We adopted a non-parametric approach requiring very few assumptions about the probability distributions that scales well as shown in our large-scale study. The entire process of computing similarities and the embedding takes less than few hours for all subjects (Python implementation). The experimental results showed that even projection on a two dimensional space can capture the continuum of the disease. This was evaluated quantitatively by predicting two clinical scores, none of which are derived from images, thus validating the benefits of the similarity-based method in characterizing the underlying disease process. Our approach can be used in longitudinal analysis to study disease exacerbation since we can associate coordinates in the embedding space to the clinical phenotype. Although we focus on COPD, our approach can be widely used in other scenarios particularly for heterogeneous diseases and when the bag-of-words model applies.

References

1. Batmanghelich, N.K., Saeedi, A., Cho, M., Estepar, R.S.J., Golland, P.: Generative method to discover genetically driven image biomarkers. In: International Conference on Information Processing and Medical Imaging, vol. 17 (1), pp. 30–42 (2015)
2. Castaldi, P.J., San José Estépar, R., Mendoza, C.S., Hersh, C.P., Laird, N., Crapo, J.D., Lynch, D.A., Silverman, E.K., Washko, G.R.: Distinct quantitative computed tomography emphysema patterns are associated with physiology and function in smokers. Am. J. Respir. Crit. Care Med. **188**(9), 1083–1090 (2013)

3. Chang, B., Kruger, U., Kustra, R., Zhang, J.: Canonical correlation analysis based on hilbert-schmidt independence criterion and centered kernel target alignment. In: Proceedings of the 30th International Conference on Machine Learning, pp. 316–324 (2013)
4. Chen, Y., Garcia, E.K., Gupta, M.R., Rahimi, A., Cazzanti, L.: Similarity-based classification: concepts and algorithms. J. Mach. Learn. Res. 10, 747–776 (2009)
5. Gerber, S., Tasdizen, T., Joshi, S., Whitaker, R.: On the manifold structure of the space of brain images. Med. Image Comput. Comput. Assist. Interv. 12(Pt 1), 305–312 (2009)
6. Hamm, J., Ye, D.H., Verma, R., Davatzikos, C.: Gram: a framework for geodesic registration on anatomical manifolds. Med. Image Anal. 14(5), 633–642 (2010)
7. Holzer, M., Donner, R.: Over-segmentation of 3D medical image volumes based on monogenic cues. In: CVWW (January 2014), pp. 35–42 (2014)
8. Liu, K., Skibbe, H., Schmidt, T., Blein, T., Palme, K., Brox, T., Ronneberger, O.: Rotation-invariant hog descriptors using fourier analysis in polar and spherical coordinates. Int. J. Comput. Vis. 106(3), 342–364 (2014)
9. Loftsgaarden, D.O., Quesenberry, C.P., et al.: A nonparametric estimate of a multivariate density function. Anna. Math. Stat. 36(3), 1049–1051 (1965)
10. Lynch, D.A.: Progress in imaging copd, 2004–2014. J. COPD Found. Chronic Obstructive Pulm. Dis. 1(2), 155–165 (2014)
11. Lynch, D.A., Al-Qaisi, M.A.: Quantitative computed tomography in chronic obstructive pulmonary disease. J. Thorac. Imaging 28(5), 284–290 (2013)
12. Muja, M., Lowe, D.G.: Scalable nearest neighbour algorithms for high dimensional data. IEEE Trans. Pattern Anal. Mach. Intell. 36(11), 2227–2240 (2014)
13. Regan, E.A., Hokanson, J.E., Murphy, J.R., Make, B., Lynch, D.A., Beaty, T.H., Curran-Everett, D., Silverman, E.K., Crapo, J.D.: Genetic epidemiology of copd (copdgene) study design. COPD: J. Chronic Obstructive Pulm. Dis. 7(1), 32–43 (2011)
14. Schroeder, J.D., McKenzie, A.S., Zach, J.A., Wilson, C.G., Curran-Everett, D., Stinson, D.S., Newell, J.D., Lynch, D.A.: Relationships between airflow obstruction and quantitative CT measurements of emphysema, air trapping, and airways in subjects with and without chronic obstructive pulmonary disease. American Journal of Roentgenology 201(3) (2013)
15. Sivic, J., Zisserman, A.: Efficient visual search of videos cast as text retrieval. IEEE Trans. Pattern Anal. Mach. Intell. 31(4), 591–606 (2009)
16. Sorensen, L., Nielsen, M., Lo, P., Ashraf, H., Pedersen, J.H., De Bruijne, M.: Texture-based analysis of copd: a data-driven approach. IEEE Trans. Med. Imaging 31(1), 70–78 (2012)
17. Toews, M., Wachinger, C., Estepar, R.S.J., Wells, W.M.: A feature-based approach to big data analysis of medical images. In: Ourselin, S., Alexander, D.C., Westin, C.-F., Cardoso, M.J. (eds.) IPMI 2015. LNCS, vol. 9123, pp. 339–350. Springer, Cham (2015). doi:10.1007/978-3-319-19992-4_26
18. Vogl, W.-D., Prosch, H., Müller-Mang, C., Schmidt-Erfurth, U., Langs, G.: Longitudinal alignment of disease progression in fibrosing interstitial lung disease. In: Golland, P., Hata, N., Barillot, C., Hornegger, J., Howe, R. (eds.) MICCAI 2014. LNCS, vol. 8674, pp. 97–104. Springer, Cham (2014). doi:10.1007/978-3-319-10470-6_13

19. Wang, Q., Kulkarni, S.R., Verdú, S.: Divergence estimation for multidimensional densities via-nearest-neighbor distances. IEEE Trans. Inf. Theory **55**(5), 2392–2405 (2009)
20. Zhang, Z., Wang, J.: Mlle: modified locally linear embedding using multiple weights. Adv. Neural Inf. Process. Syst. **19**, 1593–1600 (2006)

A Lung Graph–Model for Pulmonary Hypertension and Pulmonary Embolism Detection on DECT Images

Yashin Dicente Cid[1,2(✉)], Henning Müller[1,2,3], Alexandra Platon[4],
Jean–Paul Janssens[4], Frédéric Lador[4], Pierre–Alexandre Poletti[4],
and Adrien Depeursinge[1,5]

[1] University of Applied Sciences Western Switzerland (HES–SO), Sierre, Switzerland
yashin.dicente@hevs.ch
[2] University of Geneva, Geneva, Switzerland
[3] Martinos Center for Biomedical Imaging, Charlestown, MA, USA
[4] University Hospitals of Geneva (HUG), Geneva, Switzerland
[5] École Polytechnique Fédérale de Lausanne (EPFL), Lausanne, Switzerland

Abstract. This article presents a novel graph–model approach encoding the relations between the perfusion in several regions of the lung extracted from a geometry–based atlas. Unlike previous approaches that individually analyze regions of the lungs, our method evaluates the entire pulmonary circulatory network for the classification of patients with pulmonary embolism and pulmonary hypertension. An undirected weighted graph with fixed structure is used to encode the network of intensity distributions in Dual Energy Computed Tomography (DECT) images. Results show that the graph–model presented is capable of characterizing a DECT dataset of 30 patients affected with disease and 26 healthy patients, achieving a discrimination accuracy from 0.77 to 0.87 and an AUC between 0.73 and 0.86. This fully automatic graph–model of the lungs constitutes a novel and effective approach for exploring the various patterns of pulmonary perfusion of healthy and diseased patients.

Keywords: Lung graph–model · Lung atlas · Computer–aided diagnosis · Pulmonary perfusion

1 Introduction

In an emergency department, a patient with a pulmonary vascular pathology requires a quick and reliable diagnosis to proceed with the corresponding treatment and symptoms for many diseases are often unspecific. Currently, health professionals face a difficult task to distinguish between the different types of pathologies, such as pulmonary embolism (PE) and pulmonary hypertension (PH) [9]. Both pathologies present similar symptoms and visual radiological defects but require completely different treatments. The current gold standard for diagnosing pulmonary hypertension requires an invasive catherism procedure [11,12,22]. In addition, most patients in the emergency department undergo

© Springer International Publishing AG 2017
H. Müller et al. (Eds.): MCV/BAMBI 2016, LNCS 10081, pp. 58–68, 2017.
DOI: 10.1007/978-3-319-61188-4_6

a routine Computed Tomography (CT) thorax scan with contrast agent. The visual interpretation of the latter is challenging as it involves a holistic analysis of the pulmonary perfusion. Schickert et al. [18] confirmed that CT image analysis allows detection of chronic thromboembolism. PE and PH have similar visual signs, showing in some cases mosaic patterns due to the hypo– and hyper–perfused regions as a consequence of clots in the vascular tree. Dual Energy CT (DECT) scans have shown to allow quantifying perfusion defects of the lung parenchyma [2,13,14,19,20] using iodine components derived from CT attenuation at two energy levels of 80 and 140 keV. Several studies have presented region–based approaches to analyze the parenchyma [6,7]. However, to the best of our knowledge, no work has tried to detect pulmonary vascular diseases based on the comparison of the regions, allowing a holistic analysis of the pulmonary system. This article is based on the hypothesis that when a region is hypo–perfused due to a clot, another region or regions may absorb the excess of blood–flow, creating hyper–perfused regions [1]. Our method consists of dividing the lungs into 36 geometrical regions and comparing the perfusion of each pair of regions. In the case of healthy patients, the hypothesis is that the distribution of the perfusion should be similar across patients, presenting a radial pattern with maximum perfusion in regions close to the heart and minimum perfusion in the peripheral regions.

The selected technique to characterize these relations is an undirected weighted graph with a fixed structure. Graph–models have been widely used in medical imaging [15,17,21,24], particularly in functional brain analysis. Some graph–methods on brain image analysis consist of dividing the brain into fixed functional regions. Then, the relations between the activation of these regions are compared [16]. In this work, we use a similar approach for the lungs where geometric regions are used instead of the functional regions, and instead of analyzing the co–activation of different zones, we compare their perfusion. To the best of our knowledge, this work constitutes a first attempt to provide holistic characterizations of the lung perfusion based on anatomical graph models from CT image analysis.

2   Methods

2.1   Dataset

Experiments were carried out on contrast–enhanced chest DECT images of 56 patients, 17 with diagnosed PE, 13 with diagnosed PH and 26 control cases (CC). The institutional ethics committee agreed on the study. PH patients were taken from an ongoing PH study, PE and control cases were taken from clinical routine cases in the emergency department and control cases were chosen to be similar in terms of age distribution to the other categories. DECT images were obtained with a Discovery CT750 HD from General Electric Medical Systems. 11 energy levels were chosen from each DECT image, from 40 keV to 140 keV in steps of 10 keV, yielding 4D data with intensities measured in Hounsfield Units (HU). The resolution of the DECT slices varied from 0.6289 to 0.9766 mm, while the inter–slice distance was 1.00 mm.

2.2 Graph–Model

The lung volumes were automatically segmented from the DECT images using the method explained in [8]. This method achieved the best results in the lung–segmentation task for CT images in the VISCERAL Anatomy Challenge 2015 [10]. Only the 70 keV level of the DECT images was used to compute the lung segmentation. Once the lungs were segmented, the atlas presented in [6] was computed on the segmented lung mask (see Fig. 1). The same atlas mask was used for all the energy levels of the DECT image. The atlas contains 36 geometric regions produced by intersecting four axis segmentations: coronal (right/left), sagittal (anterior/posterior), vertical (apical/central/basal), and axial (peripheral/middle/central). These locations are based on the 3D model of the lung presented by Zrimec et al. [25]. This atlas provides adequate partitioning, grouping areas with vessels of similar size, and thus, similar texture. Moreover, it considers the peripheral regions separately, which are mainly affected by PH. An anatomic separation based on lobes would be another possibility but it is sometimes difficult and error prone in patients with strong pathologies, such as the patients we are analyzing. It is also much slower to compute.

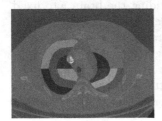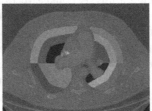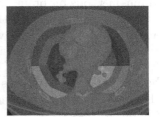

Fig. 1. Three axial views of the same DECT image at different heights showing the 36–geometrical–region atlas used to divide the lungs. The example corresponds to the 70 keV energy level of a PH patient DECT scan. Please refer to Fig. 2a for a 3D visualization of the atlas.

Every region was characterized using the first four statistical moments of the HU distribution, i.e. mean, variance, skewness and kurtosis. The mean and the variance have a direct interpretation considering our hypothesis. Hypo– and hyper–perfused areas have high and low mean HU, respectively. A region with a clot has a vessel partially well perfused, and hence, a high variance in the region.

These measures were computed for each of the 11 energy levels of the DECT images. Each energy level corresponds to a reconstructed image generated from two mother images acquired at 80 and 140 keV. However, since the attenuation curve of each component is not linear, the information contained in the

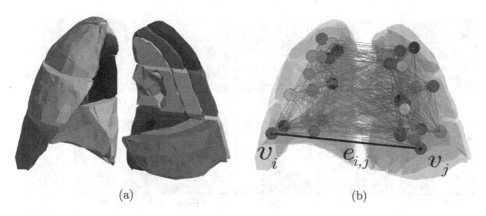

Fig. 2. Prototype visualization of the graph–model based on the 36–region atlas. (a) 3D visualization of the 36–region atlas corresponding to the same PH patient as in Fig. 1. Six regions are not visible in the visualization to show the interior atlas divisions. (b) Undirected complete graph built from the 36–region atlas. The color of the vertices correspond to the color of the respective region in Figs. 1 and 2a. v_i and v_j are the vertices corresponding to regions r_i and r_j respectively. $e_{i,j}$ is the edge connecting the vertices v_i and v_j. As it is an undirected weighted graph, $e_{i,j} = e_{j,i}$. The edge weights are defined in the adjacency matrix $\mathbf{A}$ as $A_{i,j} = d(f(r_i), f(r_j))$, where $f(r)$ is the statistics–based feature vector of the region r (see Eq. 2). All the edges between vertices are shown in light gray.

11 levels cannot be reduced to two single values. The feature vector describing a single region was defined as the 44 dimensional vector (11 energy levels ×4 statistics) containing the concatenation of the four statistical moments of every energy level. Let $HU(r)$ be the HU in a region r, $m(r) = Mean(HU(r))$, $v(r) = Var(HU(r))$, $s(r) = Skew(HU(r))$, and $k(r) = Kurt(HU(r))$. The feature vector of a region $(f(r))$ is defined as

$$f(r) = (m_{40}(r), v_{40}(r), s_{40}(r), k_{40}(r), \ldots, m_{140}(r), v_{140}(r), s_{140}(r), k_{140}(r)), \quad (1)$$

where the sub–index corresponds to the energy level in keV.

The 36 regions of the atlas were considered as a fixed set of vertices V allowing comparisons between patients. The Euclidean distances between the respective feature vectors of region pairs (r_i, r_j) were considered as weights on a set of edges E. This allows the construction of an undirected complete weighted graph $\mathcal{G} = (V, E)$, with adjacency matrix $\mathbf{A} \in \mathbb{R}^{36 \times 36}$ defined as

$$A_{i,j} = d(f(r_i), f(r_j)) = \|f(r_i) - f(r_j)\|. \quad (2)$$

$\mathbf{A}$ is symmetric because Euclidean distances were used ($A_{i,j} = A_{j,i}$). Figure 2 contains a 3D visualization of the construction of the graph from the 36–region atlas. A visualization of five adjacency matrices for each class in the dataset (CC, PE, and PH) is shown in Fig. 3.

The use of a complete graph provides a full holistic characterization of the lungs. This is particularly useful when only one lung is healthy and the other

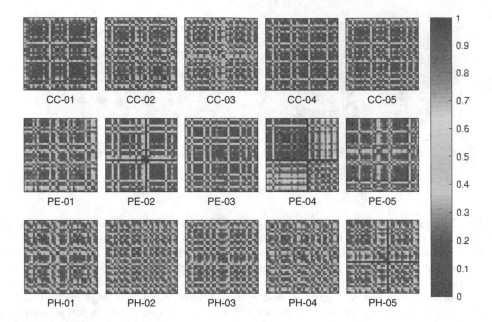

Fig. 3. Patient–wise graph adjacency matrices **A** containing the Euclidean distances between feature vectors of each region pair. Five matrices per class (CC, PE, and PH) are shown. The distances were normalized between 0 and 1 according to the maximum and minimum distance found in the 12 example matrices. In some cases, it is possible to see patterns characteristic of each class (e.g., PE–02 and PE–04 present a characteristic red cross), but visually it is difficult to find a common discriminative pattern across entire classes.

one is homogeneously affected. The edges between regions on different lungs will highlight the affectation in this case.

2.3   Graph Classification

As we are working with graphs with a fixed number of vertices, we do not require any graph–specific measure. The comparison between two graphs can be reduced to the comparison of the edge–weights encoded in the adjacency matrix. Since the vertex ordering is the same for all patients and the adjacency matrices are symmetric, they are fully characterized by their upper triangles. Hence, we use the vectorized upper triangle of the adjacency matrix as a descriptor vector of the patient. The diagonal is not used as it contains only zeros (see Eq. 2). The resulting vector is then $35 + \cdots + 1 = 630$ dimensional. The vectors are subsequently used in a 2–class support vector machine (SVM) [4] classifier with a linear kernel. The LIBSVM library [3] is used in all our tests. The feature space spans $\mathbb{R}^{630}$, where every dimension corresponds to one edge in the graph.

Four experiments are described in this article: (a) CC vs. PE, (b) CC vs. PH, (c) PE vs. PH, and (d) CC vs. non–CC, where the non–CC were composed of PH and PE.

2.4 Experimental Setup

Linear SVMs only have the cost parameter C requiring optimization. The optimization phase is not straightforward when working with small datasets due to the high influence of the random division of the patient set into train, validation, and test sets. Experiment (a) contained 43 patients, experiment (b) 39, experiment (c) 30, and experiment (d) 56. For each experiment, a global leave–one–patient–out (LOPO) cross–validation (CV) was used. For each fold of the LOPO, an inner 10–fold CV was used to find the optimal value of C with a grid–search on $C = [2^{-10}, 2^{10}]$ and a logarithmic step of 0.5. At the end of the LOPO loop, all patients were classified. The accuracy and the area under the receiver operating characteristic (ROC) curve (AUC) based on the decision function of the SVM are used as performance measures.

3 Results

Figures 4 and 5 show the results for the four experiments performed. For every experiment, the accuracy and the AUC are shown in each image respectively. Because the dimension of the feature space (630) with respect to the size of the dataset is relatively high, the performance when using a randomly generated 630–dimensional feature vector was evaluated to test the bias linked to the large feature space. The method called "Random" in Figs. 4 and 5 corresponds to 10 Monte–Carlo (MC) repetitions of every experiment using random feature vectors and then the same learning procedure. In this case, the measures shown correspond to the accuracy and AUC values averaged over the 10 executions, and are referred to as random accuracy and random AUC, respectively. The ROC curves corresponding to each experiment are shown in Fig. 5a. Moreover, Fig. 4b shows the one tailed p–values when comparing our method against the random experiment.

The best accuracy was achieved in experiment (b), PE vs. PH, with an accuracy of 0.87, while the random accuracy of this experiment was the lowest. Moreover, the p–value in this case is 2.9e−10, highlighting statistically significant results. In experiment (a), CC vs. PE, the difference between the random and the graph–model accuracies was smaller, from 0.57 to 0.79, but it is still significant with a standard confidence interval of 5% (0.0025). Finally, experiments (b) and (d) had low accuracy when compared to the random accuracy, achieving 0.77 and 0.61 respectively. In these cases, the p–values are of 0.0632 and 0.0651 and are thus not significant with a confidence interval of 5%. The small data set makes it harder to reach significance. In addition, the AUC provided information about the reliability of the classification. In this case, experiments (a), (b) and (c) had a high AUC with respect to the random AUC. When comparing PE

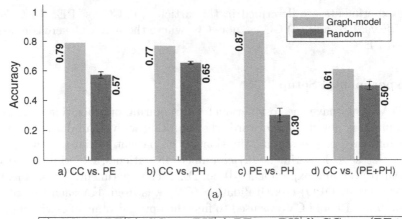

(a)

	a) CC vs. PE	b) CC vs. PH	c) PE vs. PH	d) CC vs. (PE+PH)
p–value	0.0025	0.0651	2.9e−10	0.0632

(b)

Fig. 4. Results obtained in the four experiments: (a) CC vs. PE, (b) CC vs. PH, (c) PE vs. PH, and (d) CC vs. non–CC (PE+PH). (a) Accuracy for all four experiments. The results of the graph–model are depicted in green while the performance of a random approach is in red. The random accuracy corresponds to the accuracy averaged over of 10 executions with randomly generated feature vectors. In this case, the standard error is also shown. (b) One tailed p–values when comparing our method against the random approach. (Color figure online)

vs. PH and vs. CC, the graph–model achieved an AUC of 0.86 in both cases, while experiment (b), PH vs. CC, achieved 0.73. As expected from the results, experiment (d) was the least reliable achieving an AUC of 0.65.

4   Discussion

Basic statistical features were used to encode HU distributions as regional descriptors of the perfusion. Features were extracted from 4D DECT images, containing the attenuation of 11 energy levels for each voxel and providing rich information of HU intensity distributions. Results show that the analysis of the relation between these statistical descriptors contained sufficient information to build a graph–model able to differentiate between PE, PH, and healthy patients. The 36–geometrical–region atlas shows to be a suitable division of the lungs to build the graph. The advantage of using a geometrical atlas instead of an anatomical atlas, e.g., based on lobes, is the possibility to build it automatically, quickly and reliably. Although some anatomical atlases based on lung lobes can be computed automatically [23], the methods often do not work for all kind of patients (i.e., with diseases or older patients).

The presented technique describes the relations between regions, not considering the absolute perfusion of the region. This property can be an advantage

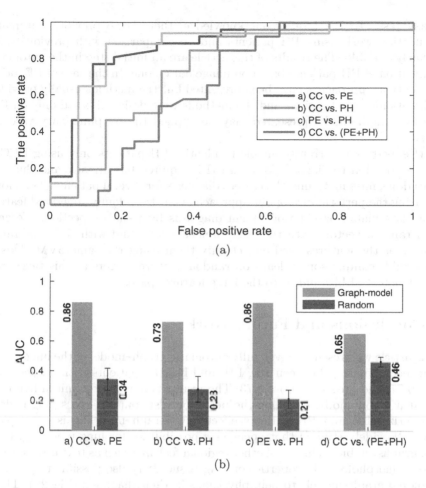

Fig. 5. Results obtained in the four experiments: (a) CC vs. PE, (b) CC vs. PH, (c) PE vs. PH, and (d) CC vs. non–CC (PE+PH). (a) ROC curves. (b) AUC for all four experiments. The results of the graph–model are depicted in green while the performance of a random approach is in red. The random AUC correspond to AUC values averaged over of 10 MC executions with randomly–generated feature vectors. In this case, the standard error is also shown. (Color figure online)

when comparing CT scans acquired with different protocols because it provides a holistic analysis of the lungs. Moreover, any other perfusion descriptor, such as texture, can easily be added as a property of a region (graph vertex).

Every patient was described with only one single vector, the vectorized upper triangle of the adjacency matrix **A** (Sect. 2.3). Due to this procedure, the small size of the dataset was an inconvenience when splitting the dataset during the evaluation step (Sect. 2.4). However, DECT is not the most common imaging diagnostic choice for PE and PH patients and finding specific patients was not an easy task. To the best of our knowledge, there is no previous automatic classification–work using PH patients and no comparison with previous work was easily possible. The results of this article are an initial step in the automatic classification of PH patients based on image data alone. In the case of PE, other classification–approaches have been presented but the methods usually provided classification of local regions and the methods were designed based only on PE, while the graph–model presented may be applied to any pulmonary vascular disease.

PH experts are currently unable to identify PH patients only using DECT. A catheterization to diagnose/discard PH is required but invasive and thus not always done, missing to find the correct diagnosis for several patients. Therefore, comparing the performance of our approach against randomly generated feature vectors is a viable baseline of human diagnosis by visual inspection. We generated random vectors with the same dimensionality and with the same range of values as the features used and classify them using the same SVM. This is a reasonable comparison to learn on random feature vectors as this takes into account potential bias linked to the large feature space.

5   Conclusions and Future Work

In this article we present a novel, fully automatic graph–model of the lungs capable of discriminating between PE, PH, and healthy patients with an accuracy above 0.77, and an AUC above 0.73. The results confirmed the initial hypothesis that a graph–model encoding the perfusion distribution across lung regions characterizes PE and PH patients effectively. Graph–modeling is a complete framework widely studied that opens new possibilities for lung modeling. First of all, graphs enable inclusion of other regional features such as texture to encode the local morphological properties of lung tissue. It is also possible to generate 3D colored graph–models to help physicians in their diagnosis (Fig. 2b). These 3D models can reveal information about the abnormal relations and localize the regions affected.

The method presented is simple and with very small computational cost and it therefore scales well. The small number of patients is a limitation of this work and we intent to further validate our model on a larger cohort. As a next step, we plan to analyze which relations in the graph best characterize each patient–class, providing more synthetic graphs for each pathology. We also plan to use the graph models to differentiate interstitial lung disease, where holistic image analysis of thoracic CT showed promising results in [5].

Acknowledgments. This work was partly supported by the Swiss National Science Foundation with the PH4D (320030–146804) and MAGE projects (PZ00P2_154891).

References

1. Burrowes, K., Tawhai, M., Clark, A.: Blood flow redistribution and ventilation-perfusion mismatch during embolic pulmonary arterial occlusion. Pulm. Circ. **1**(3), 365 (2011)
2. Chae, E.J., Seo, J.B., Jang, Y.M., Krauß, B., Lee, C.W., Lee, H.J., Song, K.S.: Dual-energy CT for assessment of the severity of acute pulmonary embolism: pulmonary perfusion defect score compared with CT angiographic obstruction score and right ventricular/left ventricular diameter ratio. Am. J. Roentgenol. **194**(3), 604–610 (2010)
3. Chang, C.C., Lin, C.J.: LIBSVM: a library for support vector machines. ACM Trans. Intell. Syst. Technol. **2**(3), 1–27 (2011)
4. Cortes, C., Vapnik, V.: Support-vector networks. Mach. Learn. **20**(3), 273–297 (1995)
5. Depeursinge, A., Chin, A.C., Leung, A.N., Terrone, D., Bristow, M., Rosen, G., Rubin, D.L.: Automated classification of usual interstitial pneumonia using regional volumetric texture analysis in high-resolution CT. Investig. Radiol. **50**(4), 261–267 (2015)
6. Depeursinge, A., Zrimec, T., Busayarat, S., Müller, H.: 3D lung image retrieval using localized features. In: Medical Imaging 2011: Computer-Aided Diagnosis, vol. 7963, p. 79632E. SPIE, February 2011
7. Dicente Cid, Y., Depeursinge, A., Foncubierta-Rodríguez, A., Platon, A., Poletti, P.A., Müller, H.: Pulmonary embolism detecton using localized vessel-based features in dual energy CT. In: SPIE Medical Imaging. International Society for Optics and Photonics (2015)
8. Dicente Cid, Y., Jiménez-del Toro, O.A., Depeursinge, A., Müller, H.: Efficient and fully automatic segmentation of the lungs in CT volumes. In: Goksel, O., et al. (eds.) Proceedings of the VISCERAL Challenge at ISBI. No. 1390 in CEUR Workshop Proceedings, April 2015
9. Farber, H.: Pulmonary circulation: diseases and their treatment. Eur. Respir. Rev. **21**(123), 78 (2012). 3rd Edition
10. Goksel, O., Foncubierta-Rodríguez, A., Jiménez-del Toro, O.A., Müller, H., Langs, G., Weber, M.A., Menze, B., Eggel, I., Gruenberg, K., Winterstein, M., Holzer, M., Krenn, M., Kontokotsios, G., Metallidis, S., Schaer, R., Taha, A.A., Jakab, A., Salas Fernandez, T., Hanbury, A.: Overview of the VISCERAL challenge at ISBI 2015. In: Goksel, O., et al. (eds.) Proceedings of the VISCERAL Challenge at ISBI, pp. 6–11. No. 1390 in CEUR Workshop Proceedings, April 2015
11. Kim, N.H., Delcroix, M., Jenkins, D.P., Channick, R., Dartevelle, P., Jansa, P., Lang, I., Madani, M.M., Ogino, H., Pengo, V., Mayer, E.: Chronic thromboembolic pulmonary hypertension. J. Am. Coll. Cardiol. **62**(25 SUPPL.), D92–D99 (2013)
12. Lador, F., Beghetti, M., Rochat, T.: Détection et traitement précoce de l'hypertension artérielle pulmonaire. Revue Médicale Suisse **5**, 2317–2321 (2009)
13. Lee, C., Seo, J., Song, J.W., Kim, M.Y., Lee, H., Park, Y., Chae, E., Jang, Y., Kim, N., Krauß, B.: Evaluation of computer-aided detection and dual energy software in detection of peripheral pulmonary embolism on dual-energy pulmonary CT angiography. Eur. Radiol. **21**(1), 54–62 (2011)
14. Nakazawa, T., Watanabe, Y., Hori, Y., Kiso, K., Higashi, M., Itoh, T., Naito, H.: Lung perfused blood volume images with dual-energy computed tomography for chronic thromboembolic pulmonary hypertension: correlation to scintigraphy with single-photon emission computed tomography. J. Comput. Assist. Tomogr. **35**(5), 590–595 (2011)

15. Richiardi, J., Bunke, H., Van De Ville, D., Achard, S.: Machine learning with brain graphs. IEEE Signal Process. Mag. **30**, 58 (2013)
16. Richiardi, J., Eryilmaz, H., Schwartz, S., Vuilleumier, P., Van De Ville, D.: Decoding brain states from fMRI connectivity graphs. NeuroImage **56**(2), 616–626 (2011)
17. Salvador, R., Suckling, J., Schwarzbauer, C., Bullmore, E.: Undirected graphs of frequency-dependent functional connectivity in whole brain networks. Philos. Trans. R. Soc. Lond. Ser. B Biol. Sci. **360**(1457), 937–946 (2005)
18. Schwickert, H.C., Schweden, F., Schild, H.H., Piepenburg, R., Düber, C., Kauczor, H.U., Renner, C., Iversen, S., Thelen, M.: Pulmonary arteries and lung parenchyma in chronic pulmonary embolism: preoperative and postoperative CT findings. Radiology **191**(2), 351–357 (1994)
19. Thieme, S.F., Becker, C.R., Hacker, M., Nikolaou, K., Reiser, M.F., Johnson, T.R.C.: Dual energy CT for the assessment of lung perfusion–correlation to scintigraphy. Eur. J. Radiol. **68**(3), 369–374 (2008)
20. Thieme, S.F., Johnson, T.R.C., Lee, C., McWilliams, J., Becker, C.R., Reiser, M.F., Nikolaou, K.: Dual-energy CT for the assessment of contrast material distribution in the pulmonary parenchyma. Am. J. Roentgenol. **193**(1), 144–149 (2009)
21. Thies, C., Metzler, V., Lehmann, T.M., Aach, T.: Formal extraction of biomedical objects by subgraph matching in attributed hierarchical region adjecency graphs. In: Medical Imaging 2004. SPIEProc, vol. 5370, February 2004
22. Tuder, R.M., Archer, S.L., Dorfmüller, P., Erzurum, S.C., Guignabert, C., Michelakis, E., Rabinovitch, M., Schermuly, R., Stenmark, K.R., Morrell, N.W.: Relevant issues in the pathology and pathobiology of pulmonary hypertension. J. Am. Coll. Cardiol. **62**(25 SUPPL.), D4–D12 (2013)
23. Ukil, S., Reinhardt, J.M.: Anatomy-guided lung lobe segmentation in X-ray CT images. IEEE Trans. Med. Imaging **28**(2), 202–214 (2009)
24. Varoquaux, G., Gramfort, A., Poline, J., Thirion, B.: Brain covariance selection: better individual functional connectivity models using population prior. Nips **10**, 2334–2342 (2010)
25. Zrimec, T., Busayarat, S., Wilson, P.: A 3D model of the human lung. In: Barillot, C., Haynor, D.R., Hellier, P. (eds.) MICCAI 2004. LNCS, vol. 3217, pp. 1074–1075. Springer, Heidelberg (2004). doi:10.1007/978-3-540-30136-3_143

Explaining Radiological Emphysema Subtypes with Unsupervised Texture Prototypes: MESA COPD Study

Jie Yang[1], Elsa D. Angelini[1,2], Benjamin M. Smith[3,4], John H.M. Austin[2],
Eric A. Hoffman[5,6], David A. Bluemke[7], R. Graham Barr[3,8],
and Andrew F. Laine[1(✉)]

[1] Department of Biomedical Engineering, Columbia University, New York, NY, USA
laine@columbia.edu
[2] Department of Radiology, Columbia University Medical Center,
New York, NY, USA
[3] Department of Medicine, Columbia University Medical Center,
New York, NY, USA
[4] Department of Medicine, McGill University Health Center,
Montreal, QC, Canada
[5] Department of Radiology, University of Iowa,
Iowa City, IA, USA
[6] Department of Biomedical Engineering, University of Iowa, Iowa City, IA, USA
[7] Radiology and Imaging Sciences, National Institutes of Health, Bethesda, MD, USA
[8] Department of Epidemiology, Columbia University Medical Center,
New York, NY, USA

Abstract. Pulmonary emphysema is traditionally subcategorized into three subtypes, which have distinct radiological appearances on computed tomography (CT) and can help with the diagnosis of chronic obstructive pulmonary disease (COPD). Automated texture-based quantification of emphysema subtypes has been successfully implemented via supervised learning of these three emphysema subtypes. In this work, we demonstrate that unsupervised learning on a large heterogeneous database of CT scans can generate texture prototypes that are visually homogeneous and distinct, reproducible across subjects, and capable of predicting accurately the three standard radiological subtypes. These texture prototypes enable automated labeling of lung volumes, and open the way to new interpretations of lung CT scans with finer subtyping of emphysema.

1 Introduction

Chronic obstructive pulmonary disease (COPD), characterized by limitation of airflow, is a leading cause of morbidity and mortality [1]. Pulmonary emphysema, defined by a loss of lung tissue in the absence of fibrosis, overlaps considerably with COPD.

Pulmonary emphysema is traditionally subcategorized into three standard subtypes, which were initially defined at autopsy, and can be visually assessed

© Springer International Publishing AG 2017
H. Müller et al. (Eds.): MCV/BAMBI 2016, LNCS 10081, pp. 69–80, 2017.
DOI: 10.1007/978-3-319-61188-4_7

on computed tomography (CT), according to the following definitions [2]: *centrilobular emphysema* (CLE), defined as focal regions of low attenuation surrounded by normal lung attenuation; *panlobular emphysema* (PLE), defined as diffuse regions of low attenuation involving entire secondary pulmonary lobules; and *paraseptal emphysema* (PSE), defined as regions of low attenuation adjacent to visceral pleura (including fissures). Given that these subtypes are associated with distinct risk factors and clinical manifestations [3,4], they are therefore likely to represent different diseases and can help with the diagnosis of COPD.

Radiologists' interpretation of standard subtypes is labor-intensive, and has modest inter-rater agreements [2,5]. Automated texture-based analysis of emphysema offers the potential of automated COPD diagnosis and catalyzing research (e.g. discovering emphysema subtypes), and is receiving increasing interest [6–10]. However, most existing approaches are limited to supervised emphysema subtype classification using manually annotated scans in local regions of interest (ROIs), which are very costly and time-consuming to obtain. Furthermore, it is unclear if the supervised classifiers generalize to other datasets with varying in-plane resolutions and scanner types.

A recent clinical study [2] demonstrated the reliability and clinical significance of global (rather than local) labeling of lung volumes using the three standard subtypes. Global labeling generates weakly labeled data that was used for the classification of COPD subjects with multiple instance learning (MIL) [11]. However, MIL has only been demonstrated so far for binary labeling of emphysema versus normal tissue, rather than to distinguish the three subtypes, and can generate unreliable local ROI labeling.

In this work, we present a novel framework to discover unsupervised fine-grained prototypes that go beyond but still have the power of encoding the three standard emphysema subtypes. Our method clusters local ROIs of lung volumes into texture prototypes in an unsupervised manner, and builds signatures of lung volumes with texture prototype histograms. The extent of standard emphysema subtypes can be predicted from these prototype histograms with a constrained multivariate regression on global labels. To our knowledge, this is the first study whereby texture-based predictions are used to globally characterize the standard emphysema subtypes.

Three types of texture features were tested, extracted from 3D or 2D local ROIs, to generate the emphysema prototypes: (1) frequency histograms of textons (called texton-based features), used in [8,9]; (2) soft histograms of intensities and difference of Gaussian (DoG) responses (called DOG2 features), used in [12]; and (3) joint histograms of local binary patterns (LBP) and intensities (called LBP2 features), used in [7].

2   Method

2.1   Framework Overview

Our framework is divided into a learning stage in an unsupervised sense, and a prediction stage of radiological emphysema subtypes using globally

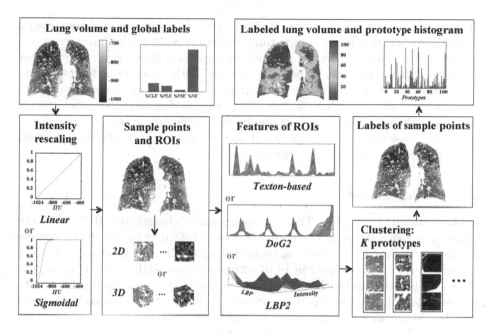

Fig. 1. Illustration of the pipeline for generating texture prototype histograms.

annotated data. The intensity of lung voxels, inside lung masks generated using the APOLLO® software (VIDA Diagnostics, Coralville, Iowa), are rescaled from $[-1024, -400]$ HU to $[0, 1]$ via either linear or sigmoidal mapping in pre-processing.

In the learning stage, texture prototypes are learned and prototype histograms H_p are built for each training lung volume.

Figure 1 illustrates the pipeline for generating prototype histograms. Sample points are randomly extracted uniformly within the lung volumes. 2D or 3D neighborhoods of sampled points are used as local ROIs, with a size of 25 mm^2 or 25 mm^3, approximating the diameter of secondary pulmonary lobules. Our target number of sample points per scan is $N = $ (lung volume)$/25$ mm^3. Since we discard ROIs with more that 50% of non-lung field, we adjust the sample ratio α so that $\alpha \cdot N - N_{discarded} = N$. The value $\alpha = 5$ is suitable for the population of scans, leading to an average of 1,512 sample points per CT scan. ROIs are characterized with texture features (texton-based, DOG2 or LBP2), and are clustered into K texture prototypes in an unsupervised manner. For interpretation, prototypes are ordered according to the average intensity value of training ROIs belonging to each prototype. Each sample point is labeled with the prototype centroid most similar to its ROI (i.e. with least distance in feature space). Finally, other voxels within the lung volumes are labeled by assigning the prototype label of the nearest sample point.

In the prediction stage, sample points and ROIs are extracted from test lung volumes and ROI texture features are generated. ROIs are labeled by assigning the most similar prototype centroid. Prototype histograms are then generated for test lung volumes following the same procedure as in the training stage.

To evaluate our texture prototypes, we regressed their occurrence against global emphysema labels in [2] on training scans, with a constrained multivariate model. Global labels H_g encode the extent of standard emphysema subtypes referred to as %CLE, %PLE, %PSE. The residual, denoted %NE, corresponds to tissue without emphysema (but maybe with some lung diseases).

In the following sections, we detail the texture features, the unsupervised learning of prototypes and the regression model.

2.2   Texture Features

Texton-Based Features: Texton-based features characterize ROIs with the help of a texton codebook. The texton codebook is formed by the cluster centers of intensity values (after linear mapping) from small-sized local patches (here 3 voxels in each dimension) randomly extracted from ROIs in the training set. Clustering is performed with K-means. By projecting all small-sized patches onto the codebook, the texton-based feature of the ROI is the normalized histogram of texton frequencies. Targeting 4 classes and 10 textons per class [8], the feature vector length is set to 40, using a codebook with 40 textons.

Note that our texton prototype histogram uses the bag-of-words (BoW) [13] model on two scales: (1) building of ROI-level texture features based on a texton dictionary; (2) building subject-level lung CT signatures based on texture prototypes. To our knowledge, BoW has not been exploited for subject-level signatures before.

DOG2 Features: The DOG2 feature of a ROI is a concatenation of four normalized soft histograms: one intensity histogram, and three histograms of DoG responses at three octaves. Using 10 bins for each histogram, following the setting in [12], leads to a feature vector of length 40.

Intensity values in CT scans encode X-ray attenuations in Hounsfield units (HU) and their range is very large. To focus the texture learning process on the intensity range of interest (lung parenchyma and air), a sigmoid function is used, as in [12], to map values to the interval [0 1] with the highest contrast assigned to the range [−1000 − 900] HU where textural characteristics due to emphysema are presumed to be present.

LBP2 Features: The LBP2 feature of a ROI is the joint histogram of LBP codes and intensity values (after linear mapping) of each voxel within the ROI. The LBP codes are obtained by thresholding samples in a local neighborhood around center voxel x. Formally:

$$LBP(x; R, P) = \sum_{p=0}^{P-1} H(I(x_p) - I(x))2^p \qquad (1)$$

where $I(x)$ is the intensity of center voxel, x_p are P voxels sampled around x at a given radial distance R, and $H(\cdot)$ is the Heaviside function. Rotational invariance is achieved by rotating the radial sampling until the lowest possible $LBP(x; R, P)$ value is found. We use 10 uniform rotational invariant LBP codes with R = 1 and P = 8, and 4 bins for the intensity histogram to match with other feature length, making the total feature length also 40 (4×10).

2.3 Prototype Clustering

The number of prototypes K should be large enough to handle the diversity of textures encountered in the lung volumes (i.e. good intra-prototype homogeneity), but small enough to avoid redundancy (i.e. good inter-prototype differences). Our strategy is to first select an empirically large number K so as to generate homogenous prototypes and then trim the set to a smaller number of sufficient prototypes (number likely different for different texture features) according to a dedicated metric. We choose K-means for the clustering task because of its efficiency at dealing with a large number of ROIs over scans.

To trim the number of prototypes, instead of testing smaller K values with K-means, which tends to decrease all intra-cluster homogeneity, we propose to merge prototypes iteratively according to their inter-prototype distance and spatial co-occurrence.

The inter-prototype distance is measured by averaging the χ^2 distance (common for histogram-based features) between each pair in feature space. The spatial co-occurrence of two prototypes i and j ($i \neq j$) is measured as:

$$S(i, j) = \frac{q(i, j) + q(j, i)}{\sum_{k=1}^{K} q(i, k) + \sum_{k=1}^{K} q(j, k)} \tag{2}$$

where $q(i, j)$ is the frequency of prototypes i and j appearing together in a pre-defined small neighborhood (here 10 voxels in each dimension).

At each iteration of the pruning process, each pair of prototypes is given a rank $R_{i,j}^{f}$ in inter-prototype distance (smallest ranks first), and a rank $R_{i,j}^{S}$ in spatial similarity (largest ranks first). The pair of prototypes to merge is the first one according to the rank: $R_{i,j} = R_{i,j}^{f} + R_{i,j}^{S}$.

2.4 Constrained Multivariate Regression

The probability of voxel x belonging to a lung tissue class can be modeled as:

$$P(L(x) = C_i) = \sum_{k=1}^{K} P(L(x) = C_i | F(x) = p_k) P(F(x) = p_k) \tag{3}$$

where $L(x)$ is the label of voxel x as $C_i \in \{CLE, PLE, PSE, NE\}$, and $F(x)$ is the voxel prototype label p_k with $k \in 1, ..., K$. If prototypes are homogeneous,

$P(L(x) = C_i|F(x) = p_k)$ can be assumed to be consistent throughout ROIs and subjects. We therefore infer the relation as:

$$Y_{N \times 4} = X_{N \times K} A_{K \times 4} \qquad (4)$$

where N is the number of training scans. Each row in Y is the global label $H_g = [P(L(x) = \text{CLE}), P(L(x) = \text{PSE}), P(L(x) = \text{PLE}), P(L(x) = \text{NE})]$ for one scan, each row in X is the prototype histogram $H_p = [P(F(x) = p_1), ..., P(F(x) = p_K)]$ for the same scan, and A is the matrix of regression coefficients with $A_{k,i} = P(L(x) = C_i|F(x) = p_k)$, $i = 1, ..., 4$ and $k = 1, ..., K$. We propose to learn A with the following constrained multivariate regression model:

$$\text{argmin}_A \|X_{train} A - Y_{train}\|_2, \text{ subject to } 0 < A_{k,i} < 1 \text{ and } \sum_{i=1}^{4} A_{k,i} = 1 \qquad (5)$$

3   Results and Discussions

3.1   Data

The dataset includes 321 full-lung CT scans from the Multi-Ethnic Study of Atherosclerosis (MESA) COPD Study [2], among which 4 scans are discarded due to excessive motion artifact or incomplete lung field of view. All CT scans were acquired at full inspiration with either a Siemens 64-slice scanner or a GE 64-slice scanner, and reconstructed using B35/Standard kernels with axial resolutions within the range [0.58, 0.88] mm, and 0.625 mm slice thickness. All scans were acquired at 120 kVp, 0.5 s, with milliamperes (mA) set by body mass index following the SPIROMICS protocol [14].

Global labels of standard emphysema subtypes are available for each scan, corresponding to the average of visually assessed scores by four experienced radiologists [2]. Inter-rater intraclass correlations, evaluated on 40 random scans, are reported in Fig. 2. The clinically-evaluated prevalence of emphysema in this dataset is 27%, with 14% CLE-predominance, 9% PSE-predominance, and 4% PLE-predominance.

3.2   Quality of Predictions

The quality of the predictions is evaluated using intraclass correlation (ICC) with ground truth global labels. To achieve a balance between the number of training scans (large enough to learn lung textures) and the number of test scans (large enough so that the prediction performance is not biased by extreme points), we used a 4-fold cross validation setup, with 3/4 of scans used for training, and 1/4 used for testing. All features were computed within 3D ROIs. Texton-based features were also extracted in 2D ROIs for comparison. We select $K = 100$ as our benchmark value, from which we iteratively merge prototypes. We report the evolution of prediction capabilities as K is reduced in Fig. 2 (all p-values < 0.01).

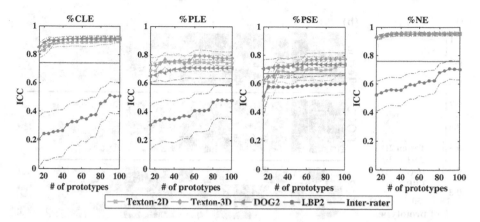

Fig. 2. Intraclass correlation (ICC) between predicted global labels and ground truth versus number of merged prototypes (dashed line: 95% confidence interval).

Overall, texton-based and DOG2 features give robust prediction that outperform the intra-rater agreement, while LBP2 features have poor to modest prediction capabilities. One reason might be that intensity information in LBP2 is compressed with our current feature length, while intensities improved the discriminative capability of the original LBP code in [7]. However, we observed that a feature length over 50 decreases the robustness and drastically increases the convergence time for unsupervised prototype clustering. This makes LBP2 less favorable in our unsupervised learning context.

The comparison of 2D versus 3D ROIs with texton-based features indicates that the richer information in 3D neighborhood is helpful for modeling emphysema subtypes, at the price of additional computational cost for feature extraction.

Regarding the effect of prototype merging, ICC values remain steady when $K > 60$ for texton-based features. Merging is capable of reducing model complexity with little sacrifice in prediction performance. For DOG2 features, the performance begins to decrease only after $K < 50$. For LBP2 features, however, the performance degrades immediately after merging, which may be because the LBP2-based prototypes are not sufficiently homogeneous from the beginning.

Note that using a high number of K, much larger than the number of standard emphysema subtypes or than required for predictive power of these subtypes, is driven by our goal to be able to discover finer emphysema subtypes. The current arbitrary number $K = 100$ will be further trimmed with an optimization metric incorporating respiratory symptoms and generalization capabilities to other datasets, which is ongoing work of our study.

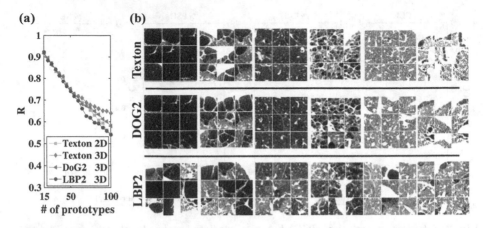

Fig. 3. (a) Reproducibility metric versus number of merged prototypes. (b) Examples of axial cuts from ROIs in six prototypes with three feature types. The texton-based prototypes are selected as the 1st, 5th, 20th, 40th, 80th and 95th benchmark prototypes. The DOG2 and LBP2-based prototypes are those having the most overlap with texton-based prototypes for ROI labeling. Window level: $[-1000, -700]$ HU.

3.3   Reproducibility of Prototypes

Reproducibility of prototypes is measured by computing the overlap of prototype labeling with two distinct training sets (by randomly dividing the subjects into two groups), in a manner similar to [15]. Formally, we measure:

$$R(L, L') = \max_{\pi} \frac{1}{K} \sum_{k=1}^{K} \mathbb{1}(L(X_k) = \pi(L'(X_k))) \tag{6}$$

where L and L' are prototype labeling with two different training sets, $\mathbb{1}$ is the 0–1 loss function, X_k denotes ROIs labeled with prototype k, and π denotes the permutations of the K prototypes using the Hungarian method [15] for optimal matching.

Figure 3(a) plots R versus number of prototypes. For $K < 50$, reproducibility is high ($R > 0.7$) for all types of features. When $K > 60$, 3D texton-based prototypes are more reproducible ($R > 0.6$ with K as large as 100).

3.4   Visualization of Sample Prototypes

Visual examples of prototypes generated with three different types of features using 3D ROIs are provided in Fig. 3 (b). Texton and DOG2-based prototypes have high intra-class similarity and show clearly distinct lung tissue patterns, while LBP2-based prototypes have lower intra-class homogeneity, which agrees with the poorer prediction results.

We also provide in Fig. 4 visual examples of prototypes that are likely to encode emphysematous lung tissues.

a) Texton-based prototypes

b) DOG2-based prototypes

c) LBP2-based prototypes

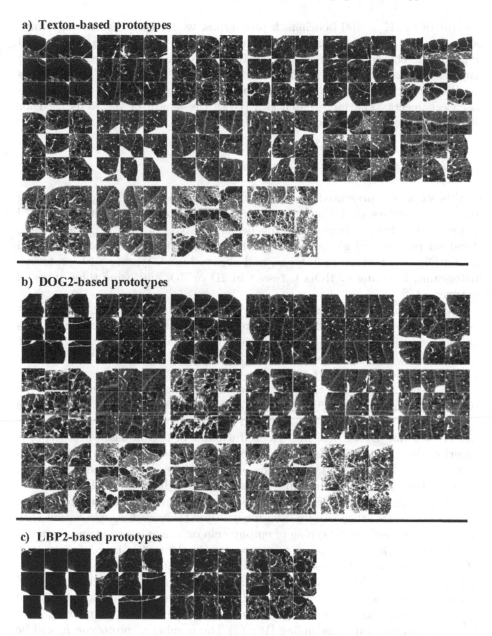

Fig. 4. Axial cuts of 3D ROIs from subsets of prototypes generated with either texton-based, DOG2 or LBP2 features and that have higher occurrence in subjects with emphysema than in normals. Window level: $[-1000 - 700]$ HU.

First, subjects in the dataset were separated into two groups: *disease* (visually assessed extent of emphysema [2] larger than 0) and *normal* (visually assessed extent of emphysema equals to 0).

Out of the K = 100 benchmark prototypes, we selected the ones for which occurrence within the disease population was 3 times higher than in the normal population. This lead to subsets of $n = 16, 17, 4$ disease prototypes when using respectively texton-based, DOG2 and LBP2 features, in 3D ROIs. These subsets are illustrated in Fig. 4 on group of 9 patches of size of $50\,mm^3$ from random disease subjects. The large patch size (twice the length of the ROIs used for prototype generation) is used to reveal the presence of nearby lung borders.

4   Conclusions

In this work, we presented a novel framework to generate unsupervised lung texture prototypes that can be used to predict the overall extent of standard emphysema subtypes from a heterogeneous database of lung CT scans, using standard radiological global labels as the ground truth. We cluster unlabeled local ROIs into texture prototypes, and encode lung CT scans with prototype histograms. Labeling of ROIs is tested in 2D or 3D, and using three types of features.

The intraclass correlations between prediction and ground truth labeling indicate that texton and DOG2 features are capable of learning homogenous prototypes and lead to very robust predictions of standard emphysema labels that outperform the inter-rater agreement, while LBP2 feature is less discriminative (at least with similar feature vector length).

We tested model reduction via prototype merging based on inter-prototype distance and spatial co-occurrence. Results show that robust prediction can be achieved with at least $K = 60$ merged prototypes for texton-based features and $K = 50$ for DOG2 features. Reproducibility of texton-based prototypes is superior when $K > 60$. These homogeneous and reproducible texture prototypes show potential in new interpretations of lung CT scans with finer subtyping. Since texture prototypes link image analysis-based discovery with radiological prior knowledge, and enable automated labeling of lung volumes and generation of scan signatures, they can be used for multiple tasks such as correlation with omic measures, sub-phenotyping of emphysema or image indexing and retrieval. Our future work will focus on two aspects: (1) As texton-based feature and DOG2 feature both demonstrated good capability at discovering lung texture prototypes, we would like to explore their combination to boost robustness and discovery power, which can be achieved by either feature concatenation followed by feature dimension reduction (to reduce the computational complexity, as in [9]), or post-clustering ensembling [16]; (2) The number of prototype K will be further trimmed to find clinically significant sub-categories of emphysema, with an optimization metric incorporating clinical data and generalization capability.

Acknowledgements. Funding provided by NIH/NHLBI R01-HL121270, R01-HL077612, RC1-HL100543, R01-HL093081 and N01-HC095159 through N01-HC-95169, UL1-RR-024156 and UL1-RR-025005.

References

1. Global Strategy for the Diagnosis, Management and Prevention of COPD, Global Initiative for Chronic Obstructive Lung Disease (GOLD) (2016). http://www.goldcopd.org/

2. Smith, B.M., Austin, J.H., Newell, J.D., D'Souza, B.M., Rozenshtein, A., Hoffman, E.A., Ahmed, F., Barr, R.G.: Pulmonary emphysema subtypes on computed tomography: the MESA COPD study. Am. J. Med. **127**(1), 94.e7–94.e23 (2014)

3. Dahl, M., Tybjaerg-Hansen, A., Lange, P., Vestbo, J., Nordestgaard, B.G.: Change in lung function and morbidity from chronic obstructive pulmonary disease in alpha1-antitrypsin MZ heterozygotes: a longitudinal study of the general population. Ann. Intern. Med. **136**(4), 270–279 (2002)

4. Shapiro, S.D.: Evolving concepts in the pathogenesis of chronic obstructive pulmonary disease. Clin. Chest Med. **21**(4), 621–632 (2000)

5. Barr, R.G., Berkowitz, E.A., Bigazzi, F., Bode, F., Bon, J., Bowler, R.P., Chiles, C., Crapo, J.D., Criner, G.J., Curtis, J.L.: A combined pulmonary-radiology workshop for visual evaluation of COPD: study design, chest CT findings and concordance with quantitative evaluation. COPD **9**(2), 151–159 (2012)

6. Xu, Y., Sonka, M., McLennan, G., Guo, J., Hoffman, E.: MDCT-based 3-D texture classification of emphysema and early smoking related lung pathologies. IEEE Trans. Med. Imaging **25**(4), 464–475 (2006)

7. Srensen, L., Shaker, S.B., De Bruijne, M.: Quantitative analysis of pulmonary emphysema using local binary patterns. IEEE Trans. Med. Imaging **29**(2), 559–569 (2010)

8. Gangeh, M.J., Sørensen, L., Shaker, S.B., Kamel, M.S., Bruijne, M., Loog, M.: A texton-based approach for the classification of lung parenchyma in CT images. In: Jiang, T., Navab, N., Pluim, J.P.W., Viergever, M.A. (eds.) MICCAI 2010. LNCS, vol. 6363, pp. 595–602. Springer, Heidelberg (2010). doi:10.1007/978-3-642-15711-0_74

9. Asherov, M., Diamant, I., Greenspan, H.: Lung texture classification using bag of visual words. In: SPIE Medical Imaging, pp. 90352K–90352K-8. International Society for Optics and Photonics (2014)

10. Depeursinge, A., Foncubierta-Rodriguez, A., Van De Ville, D., Mller, H.: Three-dimensional solid texture analysis in biomedical imaging: review and opportunities. Med. Image Anal. **18**(1), 176–196 (2014)

11. Cheplygina, V., Sørensen, L., Tax, D.M.J., Bruijne, M., Loog, M.: Label stability in multiple instance learning. In: Navab, N., Hornegger, J., Wells, W.M., Frangi, A.F. (eds.) MICCAI 2015. LNCS, vol. 9349, pp. 539–546. Springer, Cham (2015). doi:10.1007/978-3-319-24553-9_66

12. Hame, Y., Angelini, E.D., Parikh, M.A., Smith, B.M., Hoffman, E.A., Barr, R.G., Laine, A.F.: Sparse sampling and unsupervised learning of lung texture patterns in pulmonary emphysema: MESA COPD study. In: IEEE 12th International Symposium on Biomedical Imaging (ISBI), pp. 109–113. IEEE (2015)

13. Csurka, G., Dance, C., Fan, L., Willamowski, J., Bray, C.: Visual categorization with bags of keypoints. In: Workshop on Statistical Learning in Computer Vision, vol. 1, pp. 1–2. ECCV (2004)

14. Sieren, J.P., Newell Jr., J.D., Barr, R.G., Bleecker, E.R., Burnette, N., Carretta, E.E., Couper, D., Goldin, J., Guo, J., Han, M.K.: SPIROMICS protocol for multicenter quantitative CT to phenotype the lungs. Am. J. Respir. Crit. Care Med. **194**(7), 794–806 (2016)

15. Roth, V., Lange, T., Braun, M., Buhmann, J.: A resampling approach to cluster validation. In: Härdle, W., Rönz, B. (eds.) Compstat, pp. 123–128. Physica, Heidelberg (2002)
16. Lopez-Sastre, R.J.: Unsupervised robust feature-based partition ensembling to discover categories. In: Proceedings of the IEEE Conference on Computer Vision and Pattern Recognition Workshops, pp. 114–122 (2016)

MCV Workshop: Segmentation, Detection, and Classification

Automatic Segmentation of Abdominal MRI Using Selective Sampling and Random Walker

Janine Thoma[1(✉)], Firat Ozdemir[2], and Orcun Goksel[2]

[1] Computer Vision Lab, ETH Zurich, Zürich, Switzerland
jthoma@vision.ee.ethz.ch
[2] Computer-assisted Applications in Medicine, ETH Zurich, Zürich, Switzerland

Abstract. MRI segmentation is a challenging task due to low anatomical contrast and large inter-patient variation. We propose a feature-driven automatic segmentation framework, combining voxel-wise classification with a Random-Walker (RW) based spatial regularization. Typically, such steps are treated independently, i.e. classification outcome is maximized without taking into account the regularization to follow. Herein we present a method for selective sampling of training patches, in view of the posterior spatial regularization. This aims to concentrate training samples near desired anatomical boundaries, around which the gain from a subsequent RW regularization will potentially be minimal. This trades off a lower classification accuracy for a higher joint segmentation performance. We compare our proposed sampling strategy to conventional uniform sampling on 20 full-body MR T1 scans from the VISCERAL dataset, both with RW and Markov Random Fields regularizations, showing Dice improvements of up to 12× with the proposed approach.

1 Introduction

Segmentation of abdominal organs in medical images plays an important role in therapy planning and diagnosis. In the clinics, manual segmentation is currently still a common practice; leading to long processing times, subjectivity in the resulting segmentations, and high time and cost expenditure of trained physicians. Therefore, there is a need and significant interest for reliable automatic segmentation methods. In recent years a number of multi-organ segmentation methods have achieved promising results for both contrast-enhanced and non-contrast-enhanced computed tomography (CT), e.g. [1–7]. The majority of these methods use a form of multi-atlas segmentation [1,2,4,6,8]. Alternatively, in [5] multi-boost learning and statistical shape models are used, and in [7] active appearance models, live-wires and graph-cuts are used.

Unlike CT, magnetic resonance imaging (MRI) does not use ionizing radiation for data acquisition, making it an attractive alternative where applicable. Its segmentation, however, is a challenging task due to high variability in anatomy appearance, low contrast across structures, and large inter-patient and inter-scan variation. Thus, state-of-the-art in abdominal MRI segmentation is also

© Springer International Publishing AG 2017
H. Müller et al. (Eds.): MCV/BAMBI 2016, LNCS 10081, pp. 83–93, 2017.
DOI: 10.1007/978-3-319-61188-4_8

often significantly inferior to that of CT segmentation. In [9], an MRI multi-organ segmentation method is presented by combining kernel graph-cuts with shape-priors. The multi-atlas segmentation methods in [3,4] are invariant to image modality and thus have been evaluated also on MR images. Nevertheless, these results for MRI are not satisfactory for most clinical applications.

Typically, methods developed for MRI segmentation are optimized for one specific abdominal organ, structure, or condition. One example of specialized segmentation is [10], which proposes a method for renal compartment segmentation. Another example is the unsupervised myocardial segmentation presented in [11]. Some of these methods exploit the characteristics of a specific organ appearance or MR acquisition type such as DCE-MRI in [10] or CINE/CP-BOLD in [11]. Nevertheless, there are not many techniques that apply to the problem of multi-organ abdominal MRI segmentation with high accuracy.

In this paper, we propose an automatic multi-organ segmentation method for abdominal organs, which we test on unenhanced full-body T1 MRI from the VISCERAL Anatomy organ segmentation dataset [12]. Our method consists of random forest (RF) [13] based voxel classification followed by random walker (RW) based spatial regularization. The main contribution of this paper lies in the holistic analysis of a selective sampling strategy for classifier training, considering the subsequent spatial regularization.

2   Methods

2.1   Features

For training and applying the classification, we extract image features that encode absolute normalized positions, statistical properties, anisotropic properties, and spatial neighborhood information of anatomical structures. Prior to feature extraction, we normalize all MRI intensity ranges to $[0, 1]$, where 1 is assigned to the mean of the highest 5% intensity values of each MR image. The features are explained in detail below.

Location Features. Spatial position of each segmented voxel in three axes, normalized within the given volume, yield 3 location features.

Intensity Features. We extract statistical intensity features from cubic patches with edge length τ_{int} centered at each voxel. We compute intensity mean at two different τ_{int} scales, as well as variance, skewness, and kurtosis at a single τ_{int} scale, yielding a total of 5 intensity features.

Texture and Curvature Maps. Using the image itself (hereafter called the intensity map M_{int}) we extract texture and curvature maps as in [14].

The texture map M_{tex} is generated through convolution of the MRI volume with Gabor filters, which are realized as a combination of a Gaussian filter and a complex sinusoid. The parameters of this texture filter are filter frequency f_{tex}, filter orientation ψ_{tex}, horizontal variance $\sigma_{\text{tex,h}}$, and vertical variance $\sigma_{\text{tex,v}}$. We include M_{tex} as a dimension to our feature space.

For a gray-scale 3D MRI volume, curvature is calculated as the divergence of the normalized intensity gradient. Due to high noise sensitivity of the divergence operation, the intensity map is initially smoothed with a Gaussian kernel with variance σ_{curv}, followed by the removal of gradient values with magnitude smaller than a threshold τ_{curv}. The curvature map M_{curv} is then calculated as the divergence of this smoothed volume.

Anisotropy Features. Anisotropy along an orientation can provide discriminant information. Thus, we compute the anisotropy of both M_{tex} and M_{curv} in the main 7 orientations in 3D (i.e., 4 diagonal and 3 along main axes) using entropy as:

$$\text{ani}^d = -\sum_\gamma p_\gamma^d \log p_\gamma^d \tag{1}$$

where p_γ^d is the probability distribution of a texture or curvature value γ within neighborhood $\mathcal{N}_d$ with direction $d \in \{1, .., 7\}$; thus creating 14 features.

Context Features. The presence of one anatomical structure usually allows for the inference of its neighboring structures. In order to capitalize on the regularity of spatial relationships within the human body, we use context features as shifts of intensity, texture and curvature maps in a total of 14 directions (i.e., 8 diagonal and 6 for the main three axes). In order to represent information from a neighborhood of voxels rather than one single point, the image map is initially averaged over a $\mu \times \mu \times \mu$ neighborhood. Context features are extracted from all image maps (M_{int}, M_{tex}, and M_{curv}) at multiple scales of shifts (η_{cont}) around a given center voxel, such that both proximal and distant anatomical relationships can be captured, resulting in a total of (14 directions $\times$ 3 maps $\times$ 3 shifts $=$) 126 context features.

The above lead to a total number of 149 features, a sample subset of which is shown in Fig. 1.

2.2   Sampling

In order to alleviate any bias, an equal number of foreground and background voxels is often sampled for classifier training. However, for full-body MRI volumes, there exist a severe imbalance between the numbers of foreground and background voxels. Conventionally, uniform sampling (UnS) is used, where sample locations are determined with a uniform probability, as illustrated in Fig. 2a. While UnS aims at maximizing classification accuracy, it is not optimal with regard to the final segmentation, as it puts undue emphasis on correctly classifying irrelevant regions further away from the foreground structure; potentially, at the cost of classification accuracy around the anatomical borders, where accuracy is often needed. We therefore choose a sampling approach which is more apt to capturing relevant information needed for the exact delineation of an anatomical structure. We refer to this approach as selective sampling (SeS). In SeS, foreground and background samples are chosen with a probability of

$$p(x) = \frac{1}{\alpha} \exp\left(-x/\beta_{SeS}\right) \tag{2}$$

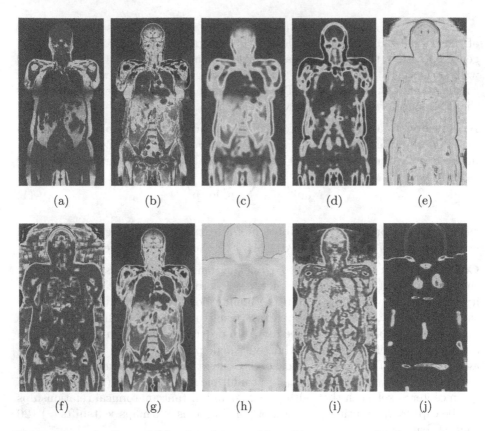

Fig. 1. Example slices of (a) original image M_{int}, (b) mean intensity ($\tau_{int} = 2\,\mathrm{mm}$), (c) mean intensity ($\tau_{int} = 20\,\mathrm{mm}$), (d) intensity variance ($\tau_{int} = 20\,\mathrm{mm}$), (e) intensity skewness ($\tau_{int} = 20\,\mathrm{mm}$), (f) intensity kurtosis ($\tau_{int} = 20\,\mathrm{mm}$), (g) texture map M_{tex}, (h) curvature map M_{curv}, (i) texture anisotropy, and (j) curvature anisotropy.

where α is a normalizing factor, x is the distance to the target structure border and β_{SeS} regulates the exponential decay. Figures 2b and c show examples of SeS sample locations for kidney for two different numbers of total samples (n_s).

2.3   Automatic ROI Selection

While learning algorithms can be highly accurate within a local region-of-interest (ROI), with regard to large fields of view, atlas-based segmentation often has the advantage of reliably detecting the approximate position of an organ (leveraging the info from a larger region and hence the entire anatomical appearance). To leverage such approximate localization in our framework, we use a multi-atlas registration framework to transfer atlas annotations to define a ROI for the subsequent classification to work. We use an MRF-based registration approach as in [8]. For a given testing MRI volume, we register several training MR volumes.

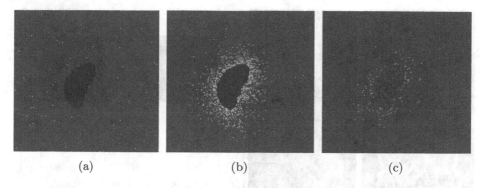

(a)   (b)   (c)

Fig. 2. Cropped example slices of (a) UnS locations with $n_s = 6000$, (b) SeS locations with $n_s = 6000$, and (c) SeS locations with $n_s = 600$. Red pixels indicate sampled foreground locations, while green indicates sampled background. Note that in (a) many green dots are out of the displayed region. (Color figure online)

A sample superposition of such registered volumes is shown in Fig. 3b, for a test image in Fig. 3a. Accordingly, we also combine the registered annotations for each organ to effectively limit our classification task to a smaller ROI compared to full-body MRI. For a given organ i, the ROI is determined by first finding a bounding box of size $n_x \times n_y \times n_z$ around the registered training annotations, and then enlarging it to a size of $2n_x \times 3n_y \times 2n_z$ determined empirically. Figure 3c shows the superposition of thyroid training annotations within a constructed ROI, and Fig. 3d shows the ground-truth annotation for this case.

2.4   Random Walker

Mere classification of pixels is likely to create speckled results, with holes and islands of false negatives and positives. These artifacts can be minimized via spatial regularization by incorporating the assumption that neighboring voxels are likely to belong to the same anatomical structure, such as using Markov Random Fields (MRF). Nevertheless, when multiple regions are returned as positives, even regularization cannot determine which one(s) are the desired organ. A common approach is then a post-processing step to select the largest connected component, which however presents no guarantees on the correct selection as the solution of the previous MRF problem is simply taken as a hard-decision (i.e. the probabilities of locations are ignored during the component searching of the final labeling). Random Walker (RW) instead is designed inherently to return a single connected component, which is a an anatomical constraint known in most clinical segmentation tasks. Therefore, in this work we choose RW for spatial regularization.

RW is known to perform successfully, given seed locations inside (FG) and outside (BG) the target structure. Alas, segmentation results can be sensitive to seed selection. We hereby propose an automatic seed selection method based on mean-shift clustering (MSC) [15]. We initialize n_c clusters centered at voxels with the

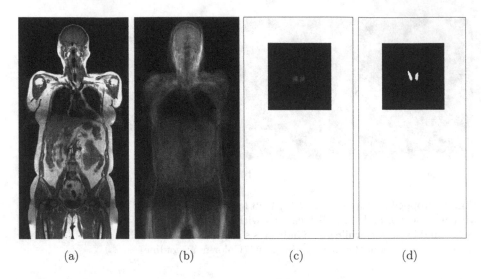

(a)   (b)   (c)   (d)

Fig. 3. Example slices of (a) the test volume, (b) superposition of registered atlas images, (c) superposition of registered training thyroid annotations within the determined ROI, and (d) test volume ground-truth thyroid annotation.

highest classification scores. Any voxel with a classification score below t_{MSC} is removed from this selection, which leaves $\tilde{n}_{c}^{(i,s)}$ points for organ i and MRI sequence s. Using the annotated organs from the training set, we calculate the average volume v_{avg} for a given organ. The MSC algorithm is then initiated with $\tilde{n}_{c}^{(i,s)}$ spheres of volume v_{avg} centered at the selected points. Spheres with mean points closer than half the radius $(r_{(i,s)}/2)$ are merged. After MSC convergence, only voxels within the largest cluster are kept and assigned as FG seeds for the RW. BG seeds are placed at a regular interval along the borders of the defined ROI.

3   Results

Data Set. To evaluate the proposed method, the publicly available VISCERAL Anatomy3 data set [12] with 20 full-body T1 sequence MRI images was used. Each of which contains up to 20 annotated anatomical structures. In this paper, we evaluated all structures with six or more available annotations. All results presented in this paper are based on six-fold cross-validation.

Features and Classification. While the method described above does not call for a specific type of classifier and may easily be extendable to other learning methods, we have used RF classifiers for all experiments presented in this paper. This choice was based on preliminary experiments with RF and linear support vector machines. We have trained separate RF classifiers for each organ, with feature and classifier parameters determined empirically with a set of preliminary experiments on smaller image/organ sets. RF tree size was set to 50, as derived

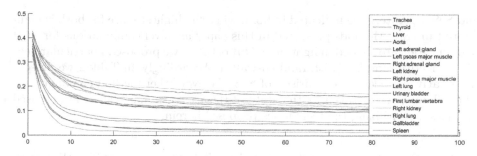

Fig. 4. Out-of-bag error vs. forest size for random forests trained on MRI of anatomical structures.

from the out-of-bag error shown in Fig. 4. Similarly, 3000 foreground and 3000 background samples were used for training each RF classifier. Different types of features were analyzed using RF variable-importance scores. We set the feature extraction parameters as follows: *Intensity features:* Mean with neighborhood size $\tau_{int} = 2\,mm$ and $\tau_{int} = 20\,mm$, variance, skewness, and kurtosis with neighborhood size $\tau_{int} = 20\,mm$. *Texture map:* Horizontal variance $\sigma_{tex,h} = 2$, vertical variance $\sigma_{tex,v} = 4$, frequency $f_{tex} = 16$, and orientation $\psi_{tex} = \frac{\pi}{2}$. *Curvature map:* Variance $\sigma_{curv} = 16$ and threshold $\tau_{curv} = 0.01$. *Anisotropy features:* Neighborhood size $\eta_{ani} = 20\,mm$. *Context features:* Averaging neighborhood size $\mu_{cont} = 3\,mm$, extraction scales $\eta_{cont} = 4\,mm$, $\eta_{cont} = 8\,mm$ and $\eta_{cont} = 16\,mm$.

Registration for ROI Selection. For multi-atlas ROI selection, an MRF-based registration framework as in [8] was used, which yields successful ROI definitions for larger organs. For some organs (in particular, gallbladder and adrenal glands), for which shape and anatomical surrounding are not good indicators and for which such atlas-based segmentations typically fail, we switched to affine transformation of the entire anatomy for the multi-atlas approach for a less precise but robust location prior.

Sampling and Spatial Regularization. In order to analyze the influence of sampling and spatial regularization on segmentation performance, we performed experiments with the proposed SeS sampling and RW spatial regularization as well as the corresponding standard approaches: UnS sampling as well as MRF spatial regularization. The SeS sampling probability decay factor $\beta_{SeS} = 12\,mm$ was optimized in preliminary experiments using a subset of anatomical structures. For MRF evaluation, RF classifier scores were used as MRF unary costs and the pairwise costs were constructed by Potts model from MR intensity images. The proposed RW spatial regularization was parameterized empirically as $n_c = 10000$ and $t_{MSC} = 0.92$.

The average of 6-fold cross-validation Dice scores per organ for all four combinations UnS-MRF, UnS-RW, SeS-MRF, and SeS-RW as well as the classification F1 scores (rows labeled as RF) prior to spatial regularization for both UnS and SeS are presented in Table 1 along with the inter annotator median Dice score reported in Fig. 4 of [12]. The highest scores per anatomical structure for UnS and SeS separately are indicated in bold, while the highest score for both is high-lighted in gray. Methods presented in this paper as novel combinations for MRI segmentation are shaded in light blue. Out of these, we propose in particular SeS-RW, selective sampling with random-walker. Accordingly, in Table 2 we present the relative Dice score comparison of SeS-RW over other method combinations, where UnS-MRF is taken as the state-of-the-art of similar classification-based methods not utilizing the techniques proposed herein.

Table 1. Organ Dice scores before spatial regularization and after RW/MRF when trained with UnS and SeS vs. inter annotator median (inA_{med}) from [12].

		Adrenal gland-L	Adrenal gland-R	Aorta	Lumbar Vert. 1	Gallbladder	Kidney-L	Kidney-R	Liver	Lung-L	Lung-R	Psoas major-L	Psoas major-R	Spleen	Thyroid	Trachea	Urinary Bladder	
UnS	RF	0.05	0.10	0.12	0.06	**0.05**	0.17	0.14	0.51	0.49	0.62	0.15	0.13	0.21	0.05	0.09	0.21	
	MRF	0.05	0.08	0.13	0.06	**0.05**	**0.16**	0.14	**0.57**	0.56	0.68	0.16	0.14	0.23	0.09	0.13	0.26	soa
	RW	**0.09**	**0.17**	**0.16**	**0.10**	0.05	**0.16**	**0.17**	0.44	**0.63**	**0.69**	**0.26**	**0.21**	**0.28**	**0.12**	**0.20**	**0.37**	
SeS	RF	0.61	0.50	0.06	0.09	0.63	0.12	0.08	0.30	0.19	0.25	0.11	0.12	0.12	0.22	0.07	0.03	Proposed
	MRF	0.26	0.29	**0.44**	0.12	**0.68**	0.44	0.35	0.62	0.41	0.49	0.54	0.51	0.48	0.35	0.48	0.60	
	RW	**0.64**	**0.75**	0.39	**0.14**	0.60	**0.58**	**0.59**	**0.76**	**0.76**	**0.79**	**0.66**	**0.63**	**0.68**	**0.45**	**0.50**	**0.73**	
inA_{med}		0.61	0.55	0.82	0.76	0.74	0.91	0.91	0.90	0.94	0.93	0.85	0.85	0.75	-	0.78	0.90	

Table 2. Relative Dice improvement of the proposed SeS-RW over other methods for each anatomical structure given in the same order as Table 1.

SeS-RW/UnS-MRF	12.80	9.38	3.00	2.33	12.00	3.62	4.21	1.33	1.36	1.16	4.12	4.50	2.96	5.00	3.85	2.81
SeS-RW/UnS-RW	7.11	4.41	2.44	1.40	12.00	3.62	3.47	1.73	1.21	1.14	2.54	3.00	2.43	3.75	2.50	1.97
SeS-RW/SeS-RF	1.05	1.50	6.50	1.56	0.95	4.83	7.37	2.53	4.00	3.16	6.00	5.25	5.67	2.05	7.14	24.33
SeS-RW/SeS-MRF	2.46	2.59	0.89	1.17	0.88	1.32	1.69	1.23	1.85	1.61	1.22	1.24	1.42	1.29	1.04	1.22

4 Discussion

Quantitative results presented in Table 1 show that, for the given data set, RW with the proposed automatic seed selection outperforms the commonly used MRF regularization. Furthermore, comparative results in Table 2 indicate that the proposed approach provides on average over 12× Dice improvement for some smaller organs such as gallbladder and adrenal gland, with a minimum average improvement being 16% for the right lung. Prior to spatial regularization, UnS outperforms SeS for 11 out of 16 anatomical structures. This is due to the boundary-focus of SeS, which leads to a large number of false positives outside the organ to segment. However, after spatial regularization, methods based on SeS prevail for all anatomical structures. It can be seen that the best results are achieved by combining SeS sampling with RW. These scores indicate that the false positives outside the target anatomical structure, caused by the focus of the classifier on organ border regions, were successfully recovered by the proposed spatial regularization strategy.

As seen in Table 1, for some anatomical structures, such as the aorta or the first lumbar vertebra, our resulting Dice scores are relatively low. We attribute this to the large amount of contextual information necessary to successfully segment these structures. Clinical protocols for aorta segmentation, for example, define the extents of the organ in relation to other structures. In such cases an atlas-based segmentation as expected performs better through leveraging the mutual contextual information from other anatomical structures.

While there currently is no atlas-based segmentation baseline for the VIS-CERAL Anatomy3 full-body MR T1 modality, [3] lists such scores for the predecessor challenges Anatomy1 and Anatomy2. Comparing the results in [3] to SeS-RW confirms that atlas-based segmentation is superior for organs such as first lumbar vertebra or aorta. On the other hand, however, SeS-RW is more promising for smaller or irregularly shaped organs such as both adrenal glands, gallbladder, spleen and urinary bladder. Atlas-based segmentation as used in [3] tends to achieve higher scores for the right lung as opposed to the left, which we assume to be caused by the larger portion of heart located on a person's left side. In contrast, SeS-RW's scores for left and right lung are almost identical.

In the future, we will integrate atlas-segmentation priors, which we now already use for the ROI selection, as a probabilistic location prior into our SeS-RW framework in order to combine the benefits of both frameworks. Nevertheless, our current SeS-RW approach stands out for high performance in segmenting some difficult organs, e.g. adrenal glands and gallbladder, even in comparison to CT segmentations. For the adrenal glands, we are at a level of accuracy comparable to inter annotator variability.

In Fig. 5a, we show the Dice score distribution of some representative anatomical structures with our SeS-RW method. Additionally, a sample segmentation

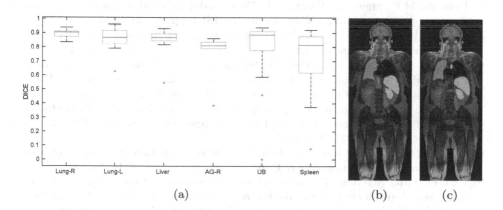

Fig. 5. (a) Distribution of Dice scores with SeS-RW segmentation, where AG is adrenal gland and UB is urinary bladder. (b) A sample SeS-RW segmentation and (c) its ground-truth annotation.

result of our SeS-RW algorithm on one case is shown in Fig. 5b for qualitative comparison with the corresponding ground-truth annotations shown in Fig. 5c for this particular plane.

5   Conclusions

In this paper, we presented an automatic segmentation framework for abdominal organs. We demonstrated the significance of choosing our sampling method in accordance with the proposed spatial regularization. While all our experiments were performed on MRI images, due to the complexity of MRI, we believe that this approach can be generalized for other imaging modalities and anatomical structures (i.e. bones) which were not part of our experiment data. Our future work will focus on combining atlas-based registration (i.e. from [8]) with our framework in a probabilistic manner to further improve segmentation accuracy.

Acknowledgements. This work was funded by the Swiss National Science Foundation (SNSF) and the Highly Specialized Medicine (HSM) project of Zurich Department of Health.

References

1. Kahl, F., Alvén, J., Enqvist, O., Fejne, F., et al.: Good features for reliable registration in multi-atlas segmentation. In: ISBI, pp. 12–17 (2015)
2. Wolz, R., Chu, C., Misawa, K., Fujiwara, M., Mori, K., Rueckert, D.: Automated abdominal multi-organ segmentation with subject-specific atlas generation. IEEE Trans. Med. Imaging **32**, 1723–1730 (2013)
3. Gass, T., Szekely, G., Goksel, O.: Multi-atlas segmentation and landmark localization in images with large field of view. In: Menze, B., et al. (eds.) MCV 2014. LNCS, vol. 8848, pp. 171–180. Springer, Cham (2014). doi:10.1007/978-3-319-13972-2_16
4. Heinrich, M.P., Maier, O., Handels, H.: Multi-modal multi-atlas segmentation using discrete optimisation and self-similarities. In: ISBI, pp. 27–30 (2015)
5. He, B., Huang, C., Jia, F.: Fully automatic multi-organ segmentation based on multi-boost learning and statistical shape model search. In: ISBI, pp. 18–21 (2015)
6. Okada, T., Linguraru, M.G., Hori, M., Suzuki, Y., et al.: Multi-organ segmentation in abdominal CT images. In: 2012 Annual International Conference of the IEEE Engineering in Medicine and Biology Society, pp. 3986–3989. IEEE (2012)
7. Chen, X., Udupa, J.K., Bagci, U., Zhuge, Y., Yao, J.: Medical image segmentation by combining graph cuts and oriented active appearance models. IEEE Trans. Image Process. **21**, 2035–2046 (2012)
8. Gass, T., Szkely, G., Goksel, O.: Simultaneous segmentation and multiresolution nonrigid atlas registration. IEEE Trans. Image Process. **23**, 2931–2943 (2014)
9. Luo, Q., Qin, W., Wen, T., Gu, J., et al.: Segmentation of abdomen MR images using kernel graph cuts with shape priors. Biomed. Eng. Online **12**, 1–19 (2013)
10. Yang, X., Minh, H., Cheng, T., Sung, K.H., Liu, W.: Automatic segmentation of renal compartments in DCE-MRI images. In: Navab, N., Hornegger, J., Wells, W.M., Frangi, A.F. (eds.) MICCAI 2015. LNCS, vol. 9349, pp. 3–11. Springer, Cham (2015). doi:10.1007/978-3-319-24553-9_1

11. Mukhopadhyay, A., Oksuz, I., Bevilacqua, M., Dharmakumar, R., Tsaftaris, S.A.: Unsupervised myocardial segmentation for cardiac MRI. In: Navab, N., Hornegger, J., Wells, W.M., Frangi, A.F. (eds.) MICCAI 2015. LNCS, vol. 9351, pp. 12–20. Springer, Cham (2015). doi:10.1007/978-3-319-24574-4_2

12. Jimenez-del-Toro, O., Muller, H., Krenn, M., Gruenberg, K., et al.: Cloud-based evaluation of anatomical structure segmentation and landmark detection algorithms: visceral anatomy benchmarks. IEEE Trans. Med. Imaging **35**, 2459–2475 (2016)

13. Breiman, L.: Random forests. Mach. Learn. **45**, 5–32 (2001)

14. Mahapatra, D., Schuffler, P.J., Tielbeek, J.A.W., Makanyanga, J.C., et al.: Automatic detection and segmentation of crohn's disease tissues from abdominal MRI. IEEE Trans. Med. Imaging **32**, 2332–2347 (2013)

15. Fukunaga, K., Hostetler, L.: The estimation of the gradient of a density function, with applications in pattern recognition. IEEE Trans. Inf. Theor. **21**, 32–40 (1975)

Gaze2Segment: A Pilot Study for Integrating Eye-Tracking Technology into Medical Image Segmentation

Naji Khosravan[1], Haydar Celik[2], Baris Turkbey[2], Ruida Cheng[2],
Evan McCreedy[2], Matthew McAuliffe[2], Sandra Bednarova[2], Elizabeth Jones[2],
Xinjian Chen[3], Peter Choyke[2], Bradford Wood[2], and Ulas Bagci[1(✉)]

[1] Center for Research in Computer Vision (CRCV),
University of Central Florida (UCF), Orlando, FL, USA
ulasbagci@gmail.com
[2] National Institutes of Health (NIH), Bethesda, MD, USA
[3] Soochow University, Suzhou City, China

Abstract. In this study, we developed a novel system, called *Gaze2Segment*, integrating biological and computer vision techniques to support radiologists' reading experience with an automatic image segmentation task. During diagnostic assessment of lung CT scans, the radiologists' gaze information were used to create a visual attention map. Next, this map was combined with a computer-derived saliency map, extracted from the gray-scale CT images. The visual attention map was used as an input for indicating roughly the location of a region of interest. With computer-derived saliency information, on the other hand, we aimed at finding foreground and background cues for the object of interest found in the previous step. These cues are used to initiate a seed-based delineation process. The proposed *Gaze2Segment* achieved a dice similarity coefficient of 86% and Hausdorff distance of 1.45 mm as a segmentation accuracy. To the best of our knowledge, *Gaze2Segment* is the first true integration of eye-tracking technology into a medical image segmentation task without the need for any further user-interaction.

Keywords: Eye tracking · Local saliency · Human computer interface · Medical image segmentation · Visual attention

1 Introduction

Designing interactive workstations for radiologists, in order to assist them performing radiology tasks efficiently, is very important [1]. It is becoming popular to use eye gaze information to allow interaction between human and computers specifically for performing image analysis tasks, as it is the most natural and fastest way of interaction. These image analysis tasks can help disease monitoring in clinics. Eye-tracking based research in radiology can be categorized into two main groups. First group of research focuses on psychological viewpoint

© Springer International Publishing AG 2017
H. Müller et al. (Eds.): MCV/BAMBI 2016, LNCS 10081, pp. 94–104, 2017.
DOI: 10.1007/978-3-319-61188-4_9

(e.g. examining attentional behaviour) such as the early work of Just et al. [7]. The second group consideres eye-tracking as an interaction tool with computers. For instance, Ware et al. [11] used eye-tracker information as an input to perform a predefined task in the computer. In a different study, Sadeghi et al. [10] showed the advantage of using eye-tracking over using mouse clicks as an interaction tool for segmentation task in general. Relevant to medical imaging field, most of these studies have been accomplished to understand radiologists' visual search patterns, differences of search patterns, and expert and non-expert visual search discriminations [8]. Despite significant advances in human-computer interaction, the use of eye-tracking technology to perform image analysis tasks in radiology remains *largely* untouched.

In this study, we propose a pilot system that uses gaze information from the eye-tracker as an input to perform an image segmentation for radiology scans in *a fully automated way.* To the best of our knowledge, this is the first study integrating biological and computer vision methods synergistically to conduct a quantitative medical image analysis task. The proposed algorithm is called *Gaze2Segment* and the integration of the proposed algorithm into the eye-tracker system is illustrated in Fig. 1. Our motivation for the use of eye-tracking in medical image segmentation task lies in the following facts. The segmentation process includes two relevant (and complementary) tasks: *recognition* and *delineation* [2]. While delineation is the act of defining the spatial extent of the object boundary in the image, recognition (i.e., localization or detection) is the necessary step for determining roughly where the object is. Automatic recognition is a difficult task; hence, manual or semi-automated methods are often devised for this purpose. Available automatic recognition methods usually employ an exhaustive search or optimization. *We postulate herein that eye-tracking can be used as an effective recognition strategy for the medical image segmentation problems.* Towards this aim, we developed the *Gaze2Segment* consisting of the following five major steps (steps are illustrated in Fig. 2):

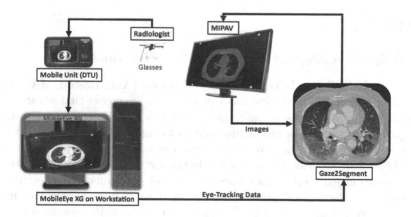

Fig. 1. Overview of the integrated eye-tracking and *Gaze2Segment* system

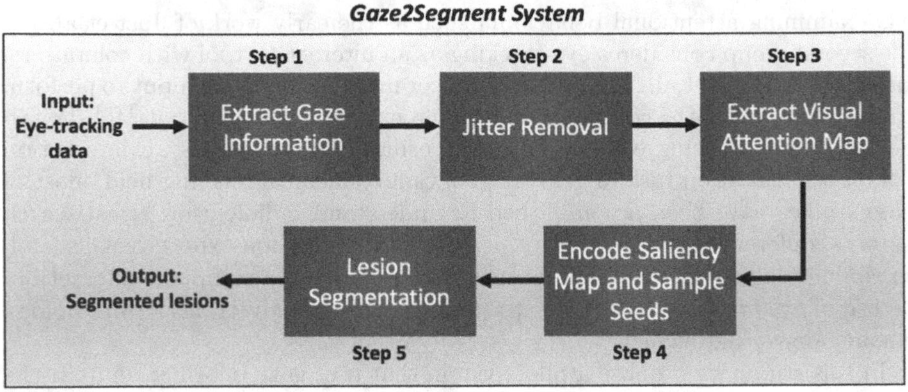

Gaze2Segment System

Fig. 2. *Gaze2Segment* has five steps to perform a segmentation task. Input is inferred from the eye-tracking data (see Fig. 1).

- **Step 1:** Real-time tracking of radiologists' eye movements for extracting gaze information and mapping them into the CT scans (i.e., converting eye tracker data into image coordinate system).
- **Step 2:** Jitter Removal for filtering out the unwanted eye movements and stabilization of the gaze information.
- **Step 3:** Creating visual attention maps from gaze information and locating object of interest from the most important attention points.
- **Step 4:** Obtaining computer-derived local saliency and gradient information from gray-scale CT images to identify foreground and background cues for an object of interest.
- **Step 5:** Segmenting the object of interest (identified in step 3) based on the inferred cues (identified in Step 4).

2   Method

Step 1: Eye-Tracking and Extracting Gaze Information

We have used MobileEye XG eye-tracker technology (ASL, Boston, MA) to build our system (Fig. 1). This device has eye and scene cameras that attach to the glasses (or an empty frame in case the participating radiologist already has eye glasses). The two cameras are adjustable to fit different users' settings. While the eye camera records the eye movements, the scene camera (second camera, directed forward) records the monitor being observed by the radiologist at 60Hz of data rate. The eye camera monitors the pupil orientations and reflective angle using corneal reflection of 3-infrared dots on the eye from a reflective mirror. These dots are transparent to visible spectrum and nothing obscures the radiologists' field of view. The data from these two cameras were transferred to a workstation through a mobile display/transmit unit using an ethernet cable in real-time. Then, points of gaze were computed on the scene video, which was recorded at 60 frames per second. A calibration needs to be performed by the radiologist before every image reading experiment to match the eye movement data and the 640 × 480 scene video. The system outputs gaze coordinates with respect to the scene camera's Field Of View (FOV) and pupil diameter on a .csv file with timestamp (Fig. 1). Once the calibrated gaze coordinates, scene video, and timestamp were created, gaze coordinates on the scene video (g^v) were converted onto the gaze coordinates on the stimulus (g^s).

Our pilot study focuses on a realistic scan evaluation by a radiologist without inserting any environmental or psychological constraints. As a part of this realistic experiment in a dark reading room, we have collected chest CTs pertaining to patients diagnosed with lung cancer. Unlike relatively simpler experiments with X-Rays, there are numerous slices to evaluate in 3D CTs. In addition, radiologists may visit the same slice more than once during their reading, including changing the image views into axial, coronal, and sagittal sections. To mitigate these, an image viewer plugin was developed to be integrated into the open source MIPAV image analysis software [9]. The plugin simply records mouse manipulations including scrolling, contrast change, and button clicks with the associated timestamp.

Step 2: Jitter Removal and Gaze Stabilization

Eye-tracking data naturally contains jittery noises. While looking at a single object, users normally believe that they look at the object steadily. However, eyes have small jittery movements that causes the gaze location to be unstable. Using such a noisy data can create uncertainties in image analysis tasks. In order to remove jitter, while preserving global gaze patterns, a new smoothing operator (J) was formulated as follows. Since gaze coordinates on the stimulus (g^s) include a set of points on xy-coordinate system (i.e., planar), Euclidean distance between any consecutive coordinate points can be used for smoothing as values that fall within the small distance neighborhood were eliminated:

$$\text{if } ||g^s(i) - g^s(i+1)|| \leq \varepsilon,$$

then, $g^s(i)$ is set to $g^s(i+1)$, where i indicates the gaze points in an order they have been looked at by the user, and ε was a pre-defined distance (based on the empirical evaluation of experimental data) and set as 7.5 mm, meaning that all the pixels within ε-neighborhood of i are considered to be pertaining to the same attention regions.

Step 3: Visual Attention Maps

There are two major visual search patterns identified so far that radiologists normally follow for reading volumetric radiology scans: *drilling* and *scanning* [3]. While *drillers* spend less time on a single area in an image slice and tend to scroll fast between slices (backward and forward), *scanners* spend more time on examining a single slice and then move to the next slice. Thus, it's a valid hypothesis that radiologists spend more time on the regions that are more suspicious to them. Hence, the possibility of presence of abnormality in those areas is higher compared to the other regions. This fact can be used to perform an image analysis task in suspicious areas of radiology scans.

Considering the above mentioned information, as well as the theory of *Von Helmholtz*, claiming that eye movements reflect the will to inspect interesting objects in fine detail although visual attention can still be consciously directed to peripheral objects [6]. We used the time information (from timestamp on the data) to create visual attention map by encoding the regions to which radiologists divert their attention more than other regions. The numerical value of time spent on a specific area might be different between drillers and scanners and even from user to user. However, the time that is spent on potentially abnormal areas is still relatively higher than other areas for a specific user regardless of the method of search. These reasons make the time a reliable factor to derive an attention map.

For each gaze point on the stimulus $g^s(i)$, an attention value $a(i) \in [0, 1]$ was created by mapping the corresponding timestamp $t(i)$ of the gaze coordinate in piece-wise linear form as follows:

$$a(i) = \begin{cases} \frac{t(i)-\hat{t}}{t_{max}-\hat{t}}, & t(i) > \hat{t}, \\ 0, & \text{otherwise}, \end{cases} \tag{1}$$

where $t_{max} = argmax_i \, t(i)$ and $\hat{t}$ can be set into 0 in order to assign an attention value for every gaze coordinate. However, for practical reasons, since many gaze coordinates may have very small timestamps (for instance, in milliseconds), we can remove those gaze coordinates from our analysis by setting a larger $\hat{t}$.

Step 4: Local Saliency Computation for sampling Foreground/Background Cues

In biological vision, humans tend to capture/focus on most salient regions of an image. In computer vision, many algorithms have been developed to *imitate* this biological process by defining a *saliency* concept with different context. The mostly used definition of saliency is based on the distinctiveness of regions with respect to their both local and global surroundings. Although this definition is plausible for many computer vision tasks, it alone may not be suitable for defining salient regions in radiology scans where object of interests are not often as distinctive as expected. In addition, radiologists use high level knowledge or contextual information to define regions of interest. Due to all these reasons, we propose to use a *context-aware saliency* definition that aims at detecting the image regions based on contextual features [4]. In our implementation, we extracted image context information by predicting which point attracts the most attention. This step combines radiologist's knowledge with image context. The context-aware saliency explains the visual attention with feature-driven four principles, three of which were implemented in our study: (1) local low-level considerations, (2) global considerations, (3) visual organization rules, and (4) high-level factors.

(1) For local low-level information, image was divided into local patches (p_u) centered at pixel u, and for each pair of patches, their distance ($d_{position}$) and normalized intensity difference ($d_{intensity}$) were used to assess saliency of a pixel u, as formulated below:

$$d(p_u, p_v) = d_{intensity}/(1 + \lambda d_{position}),\qquad(2)$$

where λ is a weight parameter. Pixel u was considered *salient* when it was highly dissimilar to all other image patches, $d(p_u, p_v)$ is high $\forall v$.

(2) For global considerations, a scale-space approach was utilized to suppress frequently occurring features such as background and maintain features that deviate from the norm. Saliency of any pixel in this configuration was defined as the average of its saliency in M scales $\{(r_1, r_2, ..., r_M), r \in R\}$ as $\bar{S}_u$:

$$\bar{S}_u = (1/M) \sum_{r \in R} S_u^r \qquad(3)$$

$$S_u^r = 1 - exp\{-(1/K) \sum_{k=1}^{K} d(p_u^r, p_v^r)\} \text{ for } (r \in R). \qquad(4)$$

This scale-based global definition combined K most similar patches for the saliency definition and indicated more salient pixel u when S_u^r was large.

(3) For visual organization rules, saliency was defined based on the Gestalt laws suggesting areas that were close to the foci of attention should be explored significantly more than far-away regions. Hence, assuming $d_{foci}(u)$ is the Euclidean distance between pixel u and the closest focus of attention pixel, then the saliency of the pixel was defined as $\hat{S}_u = \bar{S}_u(1 - d_{foci}(u))$. A point was considered as a focus of attention if it is salient.

(4) High-level factors such as recognized objects can be applied as a post processing step to refine saliency definition. In our current implementation, we did not apply this consideration.

Since we inferred *where* information of object of interest from visual attention map (Step 3), we only explored *what* part of object of interest from saliency definition. Once saliency map is created, we confined our analysis into the regions indicated by corresponding visual attention maps ($a(u)$). Since saliency map includes object of interest information, we extracted foreground information from this map (called foreground cues/seeds) by simply setting the most salient pixel in this region as a foreground cue. This step helped relocating the attention gaze exactly to the center of the closest most salient object and allowed a perfect seed selection.

Furthermore, we defined the background cues for a given local region indicated by the visual saliency map as follows. We first computed the gradient information ∇I from a gray-scale CT image I. For a given visual attention map $a(u)$ and saliency map $S(u)$ at a pixel u, we employed a search starting from $\nabla I(u)$ and moving into 4 perpendicular directions. Our search was stopped soon after we passed through a high intensity value on gradient image because object boundary locations show high gradient values due to abrupt intensity changes.

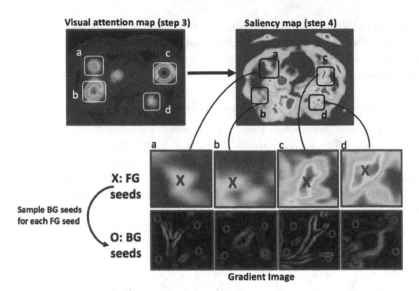

Fig. 3. Foreground (FG) regions are obtained from visual attention maps processed from gaze information. After this *recognition* step, we identify most distinct FG seed by using the corresponding regions of saliency map. Once FG seeds are allocated, background (BG) seeds are found by using gradient information of the gray-scale CT image. For each FG seed, four perpendicular directions are searched and edge locations indicating the intensity value changes are used to select BG seeds.

Those four pixels defined outside the object boundary are considered as background cues. This process is illustrated in Fig. 3.

Step 5: Lesion Segmentation

After identifying background and foreground seeds, any seed-based segmentation algorithm such as graph-cut, random walk (RW), and fuzzy connectivity, can be used to determine precise spatial extent of the object of interest (i.e., lesion). In our work, we choose to implement RW as it is fast and robust, and offers optimal image segmentation for a given set of seed points. Details of the conventional RW image segmentation algorithm can be found in [5].

3   Results

We tested our system on four chest CT volumes pertaining to patients diagnosed with lung cancer, evaluated by three radiologists having different levels of expertise. In-plane resolution of the image is 512×512 with a voxel size of $0.58 \times 0.58 \times 1.5$ mm^3. Imaging data and corresponding lesion labels as well as annotations were obtained from Lung Tissue Research Consortium (LTRC) (https://ltrcpublic.com/) with an institutional agreement. Blind to diagnostic information of the chest CT scans, the radiologists read the scan once, and interpret the results in routine radiology rooms. Participating radiologists have more than 20, 10, and 3 years of experiences, respectively. This variability in experience levels allowed us to test robustness our system. As shown by results regardless of user experience and pattern of gaze and attention, our system perfectly captured the attention gaze locations and performed the segmentation successfully.

Figure 4 shows the proposed system's visual attention map, saliency map, and segmentation results at different anatomical locations. Quantitatively, we used reference standards from LTRC data set and independently re-evaluated by one of the participating radiologists. We have used dice similarity coefficient (DSC) and Haussdorff Distance (HD) to evaluate accuracy of segmentation results over two reference standards. The average DSC was found to be 86% while average HD found to be 1.45 mm. We did not find statistically significant difference between segmentation results when manual seeding and interactive RW were used ($p > 0.05$).

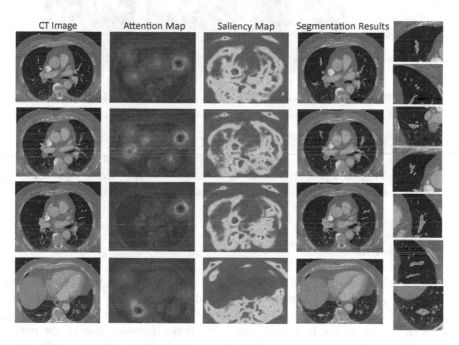

Fig. 4. Qualitative evaluation of medical image segmentation through *Gaze2Segment* system is illustrated. Last column shows the segmentation results zoomed in for better illustration.

Figure 5 shows a comparison of gaze and attention maps for two sample slices of the chest CT volume read by participating radiologists. How the attentional points are distributed over the lung CT volume is arguable based on the difference in experience levels of the radiologists. As Fig. 5 illustrates, the less experienced radiologist (radiologist 3), the larger the volume of search compared to

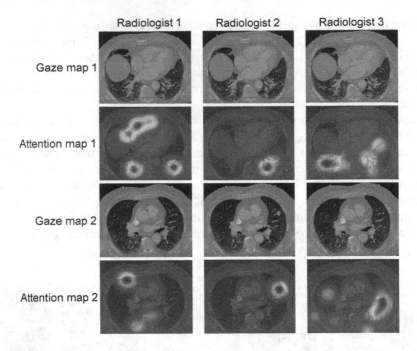

Fig. 5. Qualitative comparison of attention and gaze maps is illustrated.

the expert radiologists (radiologist 1 and 2). For the selected slices, radiologists' gaze patterns are mapped on the images to compare radiologists' search patterns in Fig. 6. While search patterns seem to be distinct in first image, pathological regions (in second image) generally have overlapped attentional points among radiologists.

4   Discussion

Since our work is a pilot study, there are several limitations that should be noted. First, we used a limited number of imaging data to test our system. It should also be noted that gathering a large number of imaging data with corresponding eye-tracking information is a time consuming task. However, due to the nature of this pilot study, and also considering the involvement of three radiologists with different levels of experience in our evaluation, the current proof of concept study with the results presented herein is sufficient for the system evaluation. With that said, our team is working on gathering more imaging and eye-tracking data to extend experiments for our future works. Second, there were several region of interests (non-lesion based) identified and segmented with the proposed system as potential lesion locations. It is because the visual attention information indicated that the radiologists spent several seconds on those regions, and our system naturally considered those regions as potential lesion locations.

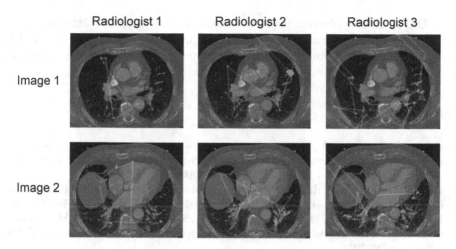

Fig. 6. Comparisons of gaze patterns pertaining to participating radiologists. Second image has district pathological regions, having overlapped attentional points by all radiologists while first image has distinct attentional patterns.

Third, although the proposed system is derived from the solid theory of biological and computer vision, there may be additional computational tunings necessary. When different organs and imaging modalities are in consideration for a similar radiology reading experience, methods presented herein should be trained and tuned based on the imaging characteristics and saliency definition. In spite of the challenges that might be induced due to modality changes our system has the potential for addressing those difficulties as well. Fourth, the system parameters such as ε or $\hat{t}$ are selected empirically. A more reliable and data-driven approach could replace this manual step. Fifth, the segmentation is performed off-line after the data is recorded. Performing the whole process online and during the reading experience in radiology rooms is the future goal. Our initial results add sufficient evidences towards this realistic and innovative goal.

5   Conclusion

In this paper, an automated eye-tracking system was integrated into a medical image segmentation process. For this task, we have successfully combined biological and computer vision techniques for the first time in radiology scan reading setting. We used radiologist's gaze information to extract visual attention map and then complement this information with the computer derived local saliency information from radiology images. By utilizing these two information, we first sampled object and background cues from a region of interest indicated by the eye-tracking and performed a medical image segmentation task. By this way, we proved that gaze information can be used effectively to address the recognition problem of image segmentation, causing a real-time quantification of radiology scans. Our main contribution is to combine biological vision and attention information with image context through saliency map. This has been achieved to perform a quantitative analysis of medical scans during the reading experience and without the need for any further interaction from the user side.

References

1. Atkins, M.S., Moise, A., Rohling, R.: An application of eyegaze tracking for designing radiologists' workstations: insights for comparative visual search tasks. ACM Trans. Appl. Percept. (TAP) 3(2), 136–151 (2006)
2. Bagci, U., Chen, X., Udupa, J.K.: Hierarchical scale-based multiobject recognition of 3-d anatomical structures. IEEE Trans. Med. Imaging 31(3), 777–789 (2012)
3. Drew, T., Vo, M.L.H., Olwal, A., Jacobson, F., Seltzer, S.E., Wolfe, J.M.: Scanners and drillers: characterizing expert visual search through volumetric images. J. Vis. 13(10), 3 (2013)
4. Goferman, S., Zelnik-Manor, L., Tal, A.: Context-aware saliency detection. IEEE Trans. PAMI 34(10), 1915–1926 (2012)
5. Grady, L.: Random walks for image segmentation. IEEE Trans. PAMI 28(11), 1768–1783 (2006)
6. von Helmholtz, H., Southall, J.P.C.: Treatise on physiological optics, vol. 3. Courier Corporation (2005)
7. Just, M.A., Carpenter, P.A.: A theory of reading: from eye fixations to comprehension. Psychol. Rev. 87(4), 329 (1980)
8. Mallett, S., Phillips, P., Fanshawe, T.R., Helbren, E., Boone, D., Gale, A., Taylor, S.A., Manning, D., Altman, D.G., Halligan, S.: Tracking eye gaze during interpretation of endoluminal three-dimensional CT colonography: visual perception of experienced and inexperienced readers. Radiology 273(3), 783–792 (2014)
9. McAuliffe, M.J., Lalonde, F.M., McGarry, D., Gandler, W., Csaky, K., Trus, B.L.: Medical image processing, analysis and visualization in clinical research. In: 14th IEEE Symposium on Computer-Based Medical Systems (CBMS 2001), Proceedings, pp. 381–386. IEEE (2001)
10. Sadeghi, M., Tien, G., Hamarneh, G., Atkins, M.S.: Hands-free interactive image segmentation using eyegaze. In: SPIE Medical Imaging, p. 72601H. International Society for Optics and Photonics (2009)
11. Ware, C., Mikaelian, H.H.: An evaluation of an eye tracker as a device for computer input2. ACM SIGCHI Bull. 17, 183–188 (1987)

Automatic Detection of Histological Artifacts in Mouse Brain Slice Images

Nitin Agarwal[1(✉)], Xiangmin Xu[2], and M. Gopi[1]

[1] Interactive Graphics & Visualization Laboratory, Department of Computer Science,
University of California, Irvine, CA, USA
{agarwal,gopi}@ics.uci.edu
[2] Department of Anatomy & Neurobiology, University of California, Irvine, CA, USA
xiangmix@uci.edu

Abstract. A major challenge in automatic registration, alignment and 3-D reconstruction of conventionally processed mouse brain slice images is the presence of histological artifacts, like tissue tears and losses. These artifacts are often produced from manual sample preparation processes, which are ubiquitous in most neuroanatomical laboratories. We present a novel geometric algorithm to automatically detect these artifacts (damage regions) in mouse brain slice images. Our algorithm is guided by our observation that the tears and tissue loss in brain slice images result in external geometric medial axis of the outer contours to go deep inside the tissue. We tested our algorithm on 52 mouse brain slice images with major histological artifacts and successfully detected all the damage regions in the dataset. Our algorithm also demonstrated much lower errors when quantitatively evaluated by performing feature based registration between all 52 slices and their corresponding Allen Reference Atlas (ARA) images.

1 Introduction

An annotated virtual 3D mouse brain populated with accurate neuronal reconstruction from In-Situ Hybridization (ISH) images is important for brain circuit mapping research [8,14,19]. The ability to reconstruct such virtual brain models and perform quantitative analysis on them requires automatic registration of thin, high-resolution, artifact-free mouse brain slice images [14]. However, brain slice images produced from conventional processing techniques are often present with severe histological artifacts, making it extremely difficult for further processing such as automatic alignment of adjacent slices and annotation of regions of the slices [20].

For common analyses of brain section images, we register these sections with a standardized reference atlas like the Allen Reference Atlas (ARA) maps. Such registration will also become difficult in the presence of histological artifacts introduced during manual sectioning of mouse brain tissues. All these artifacts can be broadly categorized either as *global 3D deformations*, which may happen during extraction of the brain from the skull, physical effects like gravity during

H. Müller et al. (Eds.): MCV/BAMBI 2016, LNCS 10081, pp. 105–115, 2017.
DOI: 10.1007/978-3-319-61188-4_10

mounting, etc. or as *slice specific 2D deformations*, which are very common tissue artifacts introduced during sample preparations including serial sectioning of the brain (shearing and tearing) and mounting slices on glass slides (tearing, folding, absence or displacement of small parts from some sections). Though most of the above artifacts have been addressed by complex non-linear registration techniques [18], slice-specific 2D artifacts such as tissue tears and tissue loss are extremely difficult to automatically detect and resolve [13]. Hence, slices with such artifacts are typically discarded, thereby, losing precious data.

There have been previous works on detection and correction of these slice-specific 2D artifacts. However, as most of them are either semi-automatic or use information from neighbouring slices, they are not scalable. For example, Qiu et al. [21] proposed to automatically detect slices with artifacts by looking for unexpected differences between a specified slice and its neighbouring slices. Hence, artifacts in an isolated slice cannot be detected and corrected. Further, such a method also requires slices to be close enough and the adjacent slice to be devoid of any artifacts, such that the difference between slices will imply the artifact. This sometimes poses restriction on the neuroanatomists who may want slices only from specific regions of the brain or want to slice the brain at larger intervals. Kindle et al. [13], on the other hand, proposed a semi-automatic method where they manually identify small tissue tears and fill them by warping neighboring regions around the tear. This approach only works well when the tear is small, horizontal and smooth. Moreover, one needs to be careful about obtaining undesirable warping effects while fixing these tears, especially when they are severe as shown in Fig. 2.

While the above techniques aim to detect and correct slices which have artifacts, many researchers try to overcome them. The most popular approach among these is performing cryosectioning of frozen mouse brain tissues [3,7,16]. The rationale behind it is that frozen tissues are much easier to slice into thin sections without tearing or significant deformation. Another technique often used is the introduction of quality control checks [16]. After sectioning the mouse brain, highly damaged slices are manually removed from the registration pipeline. Further, to aid in registration of such highly damaged slices, manual landmarks are often placed [7] or even manual initial registration is performed [25,26]. All the above measures which mitigate the 2D slice-specific artifacts and help its registration, in addition to being time consuming and expensive, require a lot of planning of the process. Although, slicing thicker sections may be a plausible solution to avoid tissue tears [2], it constrains the subsequent staining and imaging procedures. One needs to ensure that the slicing thickness is in accordance with the penetration depth of the stain and depth of focus of the light microscope used. Serial two-photon tomography (STPT), though produces artifact-free, well-aligned, high-resolution 3D datasets, which makes the registration process much easier [14,16,22], neural circuit mapping based on conventional processed brain sections continues to have technical challenges in standardized registration with highly deformed and damaged brain slices. We present a method to automatically detect and handle damages in such mouse brain microscopic slice images

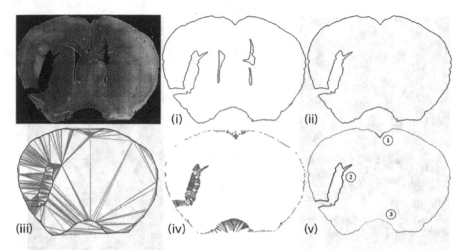

Fig. 1. *Overview of our damaged region detection algorithm:* (i). Dominant edges (MEI) extracted from the mouse brain microscopic slice image on the left. (ii). Outermost contour of MEI, which serves as the input to our algorithm. (iii). Constrained Delaunay Triangulation of vertices V & edges E using the outermost contour of MEI. (iv). Exterior Voronoi vertices (magenta) and edges (brown). (v). Three candidate damage regions whose medial axis (Voronoi edge sequence) length was above α. Points corresponding to only the 2nd candidate area were classified as damage region points as they were not vertically symmetric. (please zoom in for details) (Color figure online)

in order to achieve an accurate registration. Furthermore, since we detect artifacts on individual slices without using information from neighbouring slices, our method can be easily scaled to handle very large datasets without imposing any restrictions to the conventional neuroanatomical procedures.

In this paper we introduce a novel geometric algorithm to automatically detect major histological artifacts such as tears and tissue loss (missing data) in thin, high-resolution mouse brain slice images. We not only provide qualitative analysis by visual verification from subject experts but also perform quantitative evaluation of our method. We register 52 conventionally processed mouse brain slice images with major histological artifacts to their corresponding annotated atlas slice images from ARA with and without our damage detection algorithm and compare various registrations errors.

2   Proposed Method

Our algorithm to detect damage regions (tissue tears and tissue loss) in mouse brain slice images is motivated by two key observations. First, the contours of most of the damaged regions have long exterior medial axis creating deep concavity into the tissue (Fig. 2). It is quite rare that the tear happens in the interior of the tissue directly without affecting the boundary of the tissue.

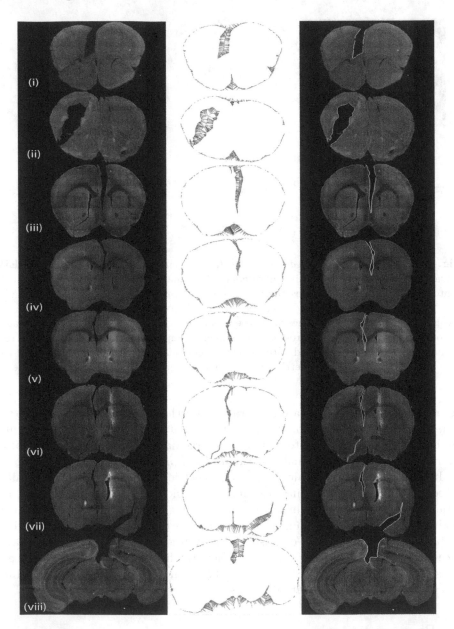

Fig. 2. *Results of our automatic damage region detection algorithm:* A sample of eight high-resolution mouse brain slice images with single or multiple histological artifacts (tears and missing data) are shown in the first column. Exterior Voronoi vertices (magenta) and edges (brown) are shown in the middle column. Detected contours of the damage regions (yellow) in all eight images are shown in right column. All the sample images were obtained from different datasets spanning different regions of the mouse brain and we successfully identified all the damage regions in all the eight images. (please zoom in for details) (Color figure online)

Second, the damage region exhibits vertical asymmetry between left and right regions of the mouse brain. It is also very rare that the same type and shape of tear or missing region happens on both lobes of the brain tissue slice.

Input. Given a high-resolution mouse brain microscopic slice image, we first compute a *microscopic-edge image* (MEI) by extracting the dominant edges using a variant of Canny edge detector. Our dominant edge detection algorithm automatically computes the threshold for hysteresis to suppress the edges with low gradient magnitude as shown in Fig. 1(i). The automatic threshold computation uses the idea of persistence of edges from the histogram of the gradient magnitude. We skip its details as its beyond the focus of this paper. We then compute the outermost contour of MEI, which serves as the input to our damage region detection algorithm (Fig. 1(ii)).

Construction of Constrained Delaunay Triangulation. Using the vertices V and edges E of the outermost contour of MEI, we first construct a Constrained Delaunay Triangulation (CDT) [5]. All edges of E are a part of this triangulation as shown in Fig. 1(iii). We then remove all the triangles lying inside the contour and retain only the exterior Delanuay triangles. As the outermost contour of MEI is a simple closed curve, we use the *Jordan curve theorem* to compute whether a triangle is inside or outside the contour [10]. If the winding number of a point inside the triangle is zero, the triangle lies outside the contour, else it lies inside. In order to obtain reliable Voronoi vertices and edges that can be used in computations downstream, we further clean the remaining exterior triangles by removing all "skinny" triangles – any triangle whose circumcenter does not lie within the triangle.

Computing Voronoi vertices and edges. From the vertices V' and edges E' of the remaining Delaunay triangles, we represent the exterior medial axis as the sequence of Voronoi edges that do not intersect the edges of the original contour of the image [1]. Since this would create many small medial axes as shown in Fig. 1(iv), we threshold them (remove edge sequence $<\alpha$; we use $\alpha = 20$) and retain only those medial axes corresponding to deep concavities. The vertices of the Delaunay triangles corresponding to the retained medial axis Voronoi vertices serve as candidates for the damaged regions as shown in Fig. 1(v).

Checking for Asymmetry and Damage Region Detection. There may be important features of the brain that may also have long medial axis, but these features are also symmetric on both sides of the brain. Hence, as the final step of our algorithm, we check whether the damage region candidate edge points are symmetric between the left and right half of the mouse brain. For this we first divide mouse brain into two halves by splitting its oriented bounded box (OBB) equally into left and right regions [9]. Popular methods for OBB estimation such as principal component analysis (PCA) [12] will fail when used on highly damaged microscope slices (Fig. 2) because the spurious edge points produced in damaged areas of the tissues images bias the PCA. Hence, we compute the convex hull of edge points in MEI and resample it such that we have a fixed

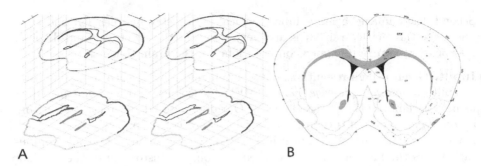

Fig. 3. A. *Correspondences used during feature based non-linear registration:* Dense correspondences before (left) and after (right) our damage region detection algorithm between MEI (bottom) and its corresponding atlas from ARA maps (top). Correspondences are shown using similarly colored curve segments. B. *Computation of registration errors:* 20 manually selected points (magenta) are uniformly distributed and overlayed on the atlas from ARA maps (background). Error between their corresponding points in the matching microscopic slice is computed and reported in Table. 1. (please zoom in for details) (Color figure online)

number of points uniformly sampled along the convex hull. We then use PCA on the resampled convex hull curves to compute the OBB of the microscopic image slice. The combination of PCA on the resampled convex hull curve eliminates the edge effects including bias due to noise, tissue damage and other artifacts caused during sample preparation.

We then check for symmetry of the candidate edges of the damaged region by reflecting those edge points about the vertical axis dividing the OBB in half and using a small neighborhood to search for points having similar normal vectors around the expected region of symmetry. Normal vectors of edge points are computed using moving least squares [17] as it smoothly interpolates the normal vectors, diminishing the effect of noise, sharp features and topological foldings. Candidate edge points, which are asymmetric between the left and right regions of the brain are classified as damage region points. For example, as shown in Fig. 1, out of the three candidate damage regions, only the points corresponding to the 2nd candidate damage region were classified as damage region points. Points corresponding to the remaining two (1st & 2nd) candidate damage regions form important features of the mouse brain slice images and hence are also vertically symmetric.

3   Results and Discussion

We evaluate our algorithm on 52 conventionally processed microscopic images of coronal mouse brain slices (5000×8000 pixels) with a resolution of $0.6\,\mu$m per pixel. These images were manually identified by subject experts from different

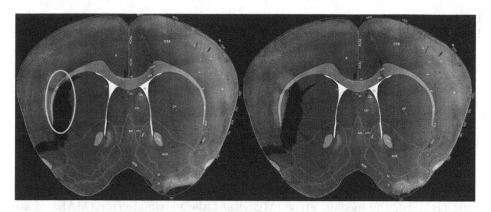

Fig. 4. *Results from feature based registration techniques with and without our algorithm:* The figure shows results of a standard feature based non-linear registration with corresponding ARA (overlayed in white) without (left) and with (right) our damage region detection algorithm. Incorrect registration is shown using yellow marked regions. (please zoom in for details) (Color figure online)

mouse brain datasets to contain severe histological artifacts such as tears and missing data. These artifacts were produced either during serial sectioning of the mouse brain tissue or mounting of the thin slices on glass slides. Among the 52 slices, 45 slices had single tears or missing regions while 7 slices had multiple tears or missing regions. We ran our automatic damage region detection algorithm on all 52 microscopic images and successfully identified the damage regions in all of them as shown in Fig. 2. Our damage region detection results were found qualitatively quite accurate by the subject experts.

We also quantitatively evaluate our algorithm by comparing results from standard feature based registration techniques when used with and without our damage region detection algorithm. Feature based registration algorithms have been quite popular in the past for registration of microscopic images [4,6,15,23]. However, the presence of edges due to the damage regions misleads and corrupts the correspondence finding (Fig. 3A), resulting in bad registration. Hence, it is important to first accurately identify and remove points in the damage regions before performing feature based registration.

We perform an inter-stack feature based registration where we align all 52 microscopic images with their corresponding annotated atlases from ARA maps[1] with and without damage region detection. In both cases, for registration, we first perform global affine alignment using a variant of iterative closest point (ICP) [24]. This is followed by a final non-linear alignment by solving the Laplace's equation with Dirichlet boundary conditions [11] (Fig. 4). The only difference between the two cases is our damage region detection algorithm where the detected damage region points are excluded from the correspondence finding as shown in Fig. 3A. For statistical analysis we compared the root-mean-squared

---

[1] Publically available from the Allen Brain Atlas Project.

Table 1. Comparison of registration errors (in pixels) with and without our damage detection algorithm after affine and final non-linear (affine+elastic) transformations.

	With our algorithm			Without our algorithm		
	Average RMSE	Average MEE	Average MAE	Average RMSE	Average MEE	Average MAE
After affine transformation	13.37	10.66	25.27	16.28	13.30	30.79
After non-linear transformation	3.91	2.53	4.36	5.51	4.47	11.90

error (RMSE), the median error (MEE) and the maximal error (MAE) of 20 corresponding points which were manually picked and distributed uniformly in the microscopic and atlas image pair (Fig. 3B). Table 1 summarizes the registration errors after both affine and non-linear transformation with and without our damage region detection algorithm. We found lower registration errors when alignment was performed with our algorithm than without it.

We have developed and demonstrated a completely automatic algorithm to not only identify but accurately locate and handle slice-specific histological artifacts such as tissue tears and tissue loss in high-resolution microscopic mouse brain slice images. As these artifacts are very common in conventionally processed slices, our algorithm will have wide applicability and usefulness in broad range of experiments and neuroanatomical laboratories. We show results of one such application where we perform accurate registration of highly damage slices with their corresponding annotated atlas from ARA maps. Such applications play a vital role in reconstruction of mouse brain datasets. Another advantage of our algorithm is that it can locate multiple such artifacts that may be present in single slice images as shown in Fig. 2(vi) and (vii). This enables and facilitates extremely thin sectioning of the mouse brain tissue, which is necessary for an accurate 3D mouse brain model reconstruction. To further illustrate the difficulty and the effectiveness of our method, we also show the results of our damage region detection algorithm on a synthetically damaged slice image with more than three tissue tears, which are deep and randomly placed (Fig. 5).

However, there are still some extreme artifacts, which cannot be handled by our algorithm. For example, slices in which the tear goes all the way through will have more than one component. Such tissues are very difficult to mount since multiple components have to be accurately placed in their original positions onto the glass slide. In such cases, our algorithm will fail as it detects multiple components, and hence we do not process such slices any further. Few other extreme deformations are folding of the tissue and overlap of adjacent tissue regions. For such artifacts, a more complicated or semi-automatic approach might be helpful.

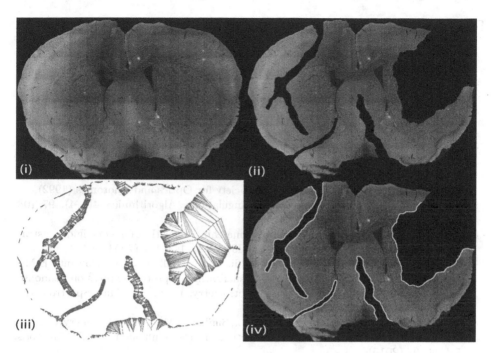

Fig. 5. *Results of our automatic damage region detection algorithm on a synthetically damaged mouse brain slice image:* To show the variety of damages our algorithm can handle, we ran our algorithm on a synthetically created damage slice image with four different types of tissue tears at different locations. (i). Original mouse brain micro scopic slice image. (ii). Synthetically damaged slice image with four tissue tears. (iii). Exterior Voronoi vertices (magenta) and edges (brown). (iv). Detected contours of all the damage regions (yellow) overlayed on the damaged slice image. We successfully detected all the four different types of tears in the mouse brain slice image. (please zoom in for details) (Color figure online)

4 Conclusion

To the best of our knowledge the presented work is the first that automatically detects slice-specific histological artifacts such as tissue tears and tissue loss in high-resolution mouse brain slice images without using information from neighbouring slices. Our robust damaged region detection algorithm condones histological artifacts that occur in standard procedures to produce brain slice images. We believe that this work will have a major impact on brain circuit mapping by facilitating conventional neuroanatomical image registration and creation of 3-D whole brain map databases.

Acknowledgement. The authors would like to thank Dr Hong-Wei Dong for providing the mouse brain atlas contour images. This work was supported in part by NIH grants (R01MH105427 and R01NS078434).

References

1. Amenta, N., Bern, M., Eppstein, D.: The crust and the β-skeleton: combinatorial curve reconstruction. Graph. Model Image Process. **60**(2), 125–135 (1998)
2. Berlanga, M.L., Phan, S., Bushong, E.A., Wu, S., Kwon, O., Phung, B.S., Lamont, S., Terada, M., Tasdizen, T., Martone, M.E., et al.: Three-dimensional reconstruction of serial mouse brain sections: solution for flattening high-resolution large-scale mosaics. Front. Neuroanatomy **5**, 17 (2011)
3. Bertrand, L., Nissanov, J.: The neuroterrain 3d mouse brain atlas. Front. Neuroinform. **2**, 3 (2008)
4. Besl, P.J., McKay, N.D.: Method for registration of 3-d shapes. In: Robotics-DL Tentative, pp. 586–606. International Society for Optics and Photonics (1992)
5. Chew, L.P.: Constrained delaunay triangulations. Algorithmica **4**(1–4), 97–108 (1989)
6. Chui, H., Rangarajan, A.: A new point matching algorithm for non-rigid registration. Comput. Vis. Image Underst. (CVIJ) **89**(2), 114–141 (2003)
7. Crecelius, A.C., Cornett, D.S., Caprioli, R.M., Williams, B., Dawant, B.M., Bodenheimer, B.: Three-dimensional visualization of protein expression in mouse brain structures using imaging mass spectrometry. J. Am. Soc. Mass Spectrometry **16**(7), 1093–1099 (2005)
8. Feng, D., Lau, C., Ng, L., Li, Y., Kuan, L., Sunkin, S.M., Dang, C., Hawrylycz, M.: Exploration and visualization of connectivity in the adult mouse brain. Methods **73**, 90–97 (2015)
9. Gottschalk, S., Lin, M.C., Manocha, D.: OBBTree: a hierarchical structure for rapid interference detection. In: Proceedings of the 23rd Annual Conference on Computer Graphics and Interactive Techniques, pp. 171–180. ACM (1996)
10. Hormann, K., Agathos, A.: The point in polygon problem for arbitrary polygons. Comput. Geometry **20**(3), 131–144 (2001)
11. Jeschke, S., Cline, D., Wonka, P.: A GPU laplacian solver for diffusion curves and poisson image editing. ACM Trans. Graphics (TOG) **28**, 116 (2009)
12. Jolliffe, I.: Principal Component Analysis. Wiley Online Library (2002)
13. Kindle, L.M., Kakadiaris, I.A., Ju, T., Carson, J.P.: A semiautomated approach for artefact removal in serial tissue cryosections. J. Microscopy **241**(2), 200–206 (2011)
14. Kuan, L., Li, Y., Lau, C., Feng, D., Bernard, A., Sunkin, S.M., Zeng, H., Dang, C., Hawrylycz, M., Ng, L.: Neuroinformatics of the allen mouse brain connectivity atlas. Methods **73**, 4–17 (2015)
15. Kurkure, U., Le, Y.H., Paragios, N., Carson, J.P., Ju, T., Kakadiaris, I.A.: Landmark/image-based deformable registration of gene expression data. In: 2011 IEEE Conference on Computer Vision and Pattern Recognition (CVPR), pp. 1089–1096. IEEE (2011)
16. Lein, E.S., Hawrylycz, M.J., Ao, N., Ayres, M., Bensinger, A., Bernard, A., Boe, A.F., Boguski, M.S., Brockway, K.S., Byrnes, E.J., et al.: Genome-wide atlas of gene expression in the adult mouse brain. Nature **445**(7124), 168–176 (2007)
17. Levin, D.: The approximation power of moving least-squares. Math. Comput. Am. Math. Soc. **67**(224), 1517–1531 (1998)
18. Ng, L., Hawrylycz, M., Haynor, D.: Automated high-throughput registration for localizing 3d mouse brain gene expression using ITK. In: IJ-2005 MICCAI Open-Source Workshop (2005)

19. Oh, S.W., Harris, J.A., Ng, L., Winslow, B., Cain, N., Mihalas, S., Wang, Q., Lau, C., Kuan, L., Henry, A.M., et al.: A mesoscale connectome of the mouse brain. Nature 508(7495), 207–214 (2014)
20. Ourselin, S., Roche, A., Subsol, G., Pennec, X., Ayache, N.: Reconstructing a 3d structure from serial histological sections. Image Vis. Comput. 19(1), 25–31 (2001)
21. Qiu, X., Pridmore, T., Pitiot, A.: Correcting distorted histology slices for 3D reconstruction. Proc. Med. Image Underst. Anal., 224–228, July 2009
22. Ragan, T., Kadiri, L.R., Venkataraju, K.U., Bahlmann, K., Sutin, J., Taranda, J., Arganda-Carreras, I., Kim, Y., Seung, H.S., Osten, P.: Serial two-photon tomography for automated ex vivo mouse brain imaging. Nature Methods 9(3), 255–258 (2012)
23. Rangarajan, A., Chui, H., Mjolsness, E., Pappu, S., Davachi, L., Goldman-Rakic, P., Duncan, J.: A robust point-matching algorithm for autoradiograph alignment. Med. Image Anal. 1(4), 379–398 (1997)
24. Rusinkiewicz, S., Levoy, M.: Efficient variants of the ICP algorithm. In: Third International Conference on 3-D Digital Imaging and Modeling, Proceedings, pp. 145–152. IEEE (2001)
25. Sawiak, S.J., Williams, G.B., Wood, N.I., Morton, A.J., Carpenter, T.A.: SPM-Mouse: a new toolbox for SPM in the animal brain. In: ISMRM 17th Scientific Meeting & Exhibition, pp. 18–24 (2009)
26. Vousden, D.A., Epp, J., Okuno, H., Nieman, B.J., van Eede, M., Dazai, J., Ragan, T., Bito, H., Frankland, P.W., Lerch, J.P., et al.: Whole-brain mapping of behaviourally induced neural activation in mice. Brain Struct. Func. 220(4), 2043–2057 (2015). doi:10.1007/s00429-014-0774-0

Lung Nodule Classification by Jointly Using Visual Descriptors and Deep Features

Yutong Xie[1,2], Jianpeng Zhang[1,2], Sidong Liu[3], Weidong Cai[3], and Yong Xia[1,2(✉)]

[1] Shaanxi Key Lab of Speech & Image Information Processing (SAIIP),
School of Computer Science and Engineering,
Northwestern Polytechnical University, Xi'an 710072, PR China
yxia@nwpu.edu.cn
[2] Centre for Multidisciplinary Convergence Computing (CMCC),
School of Computer Science and Engineering,
Northwestern Polytechnical University, Xi'an 710072, PR China
[3] Biomedical and Multimedia Information Technology (BMIT) Research Group,
School of Information Technologies, University of Sydney,
Sydney, NSW 2006, Australia

Abstract. Classifying benign and malignant lung nodules using the thoracic computed tomography (CT) screening is the primary method for early diagnosis of lung cancer. Despite of their widely recognized success in image classification, deep learning techniques may not achieve satisfying accuracy on this problem, due to the limited training samples resulted from the all-consuming nature of medical image acquisition and annotation. In this paper, we jointly use the texture and shape descriptors, which characterize the heterogeneity of nodules, and the features learned by a deep convolutional neural network, and thus proposed a combined-feature based classification (CFBC) algorithm to differentiate lung nodules. We have evaluated this algorithm against four state-of-the-art nodule classification approaches on the benchmark LIDC-IDRI dataset. Our results suggest that the proposed CFBC algorithm can distinguish malignant lung nodules from benign ones more accurately than other four methods.

Keywords: Lung nodule classification · Computed tomography · Deep convolutional neural network · Texture descriptor · Shape descriptor

1 Introduction

Lung cancer is the number one cause of cancer deaths in both men and women worldwide [1, 2]. The most effective way to improve survival of patients is the early diagnosis and treatment, since the 5-year survival rate is approximately 54% if the pathology is detected in initial stages and only 4% if detected in advanced stages [3, 4]. Computed Tomography (CT), especially high resolution CT, is one the most important imaging modalities for lung cancer diagnosis. In chest CT scans, a "spot" on the lung that is less than 3 cm in diameter is called a lung nodule, which can be either benign (non-cancerous) or malignant (cancerous). The overall chance that a lung nodule is

© Springer International Publishing AG 2017
H. Müller et al. (Eds.): MCV/BAMBI 2016, LNCS 10081, pp. 116–125, 2017.
DOI: 10.1007/978-3-319-61188-4_11

cancer is 40%, but that risk varies a lot depending on what the nodule looks like. Therefore, it is critically important to classify lung nodules into benign and malignant ones.

The enormous number of chest CT images produced globally are currently ana-lyzed almost entirely through visual inspection on a slice-by-slice basis. This requires a high degree of skill and concentration, and is time-consuming, expensive, and prone to operator bias. Computer-aided lung nodule classification using CT would not only enable radiologists and researchers to bypass these issues, but to provide effective and timely diagnosis with unprecedented social benefits. It, therefore, has drawn more and more researches attention in the medical imaging community during the past two decades, resulting in many lung nodule classification approaches in the literature, most of which consist of two steps: extracting numerical features to characterize lung nodules and applying the features to a trained classifier.

The features used for nodule classification can be roughly categorized into two groups: texture descriptors and shape descriptors. The most commonly used texture descriptor is estimated based on the gray level co-occurrence matrix (GLCM) [5]. Wu et al. [6] extracted 13 gray level co-occurrence matrix textural features and 12 radio-logical features for the differentiation of malignant from benign solitary pulmonary nodules. Aggarwal et al. [7] calculated GLCM features and applied them to the linear discriminate analysis (LDA) for lung nodule detection and classification in chest CT scans. Mabrouk et al. [8] extracted the 80-dimensional GLCM features and adopted a feature selection procedure to identify the most effective components before applying them to the support vector machine (SVM) [9] classifier for automated lung nodule classification. Anand [10] calculated GLCM features and ted them as the input of a back propagation (BP) neural network for lung nodule classification. Wei et al. [4] proposed multi-scale convolutional neural networks to capture lung nodule hetero-geneity by learning a set of class-specific features from each input scale before applying them to SVM and random forest (RF). Several features, such as the Feret shape measure, roundness, moment invariants, point distance histogram and Fourier descriptor, can be applied to shape description. Frejlichowski [11] proved that the Fourier descriptor has an excellent performance in general shape analysis. Sokic and Konjicija [12] extracted one-dimensional Fourier descriptor for content-based image retrieval. Zhang and Lu [13] extended this descriptor to 2D for regional shape description.

Once features are extracted, most classification technique, such as SVM [8, 14, 15], BP neural network [10, 16] and RF [4, 17, 18], can be applied to solve this problem. Recently, deep learning [19] has become a powerful tool in a number of areas, including image generation, annotation and classification. Deep models provide a uniform framework for learning-based joint feature extraction and classification, avoiding the hand-crafted feature extraction that may lead to less accurate classifica-tion. Hua et al. [20] applied both the deep convolutional neural network (DCNN) and deep belief network (DBN) to lung nodule classification and confirmed that deep learning can achieve better discrimination between benign and malignant nodules.

Despite of the improved accuracy, deep learning techniques may suffer from over-fitting when applied to lung nodule classification, since there usually is only a relatively small set of training samples due to the all-consuming nature of medical image acquisition and annotation. We suggest that the texture descriptors and shape descriptors derived under the guidance of the heuristics that the heterogeneity in shape and voxel values is a major characteristic of malignant nodule may complement the features learned by deep models and hence alleviate the inaccuracy caused by over-fitting.

In this paper, we propose a combined-feature based classification (CFBC) algorithm to differentiate malignant lung nodules from benign ones by jointly using the texture and shape descriptors, which characterize the nodule heterogeneity, and the features learned by deep neural networks for lung nodule classification. We employ a nine-layer DCNN to extract deep features, adopted the GLCM features and Fourier descriptors to characterize the texture and shape of each nodule, respectively, and apply the combined features to a BP neural network. We have evaluated the proposed algorithm against four state-of-the-art lung nodule classification approaches on the benchmark LIDC-IDRI dataset [21].

The paper is organized as follows: in Sect. 2, we introduce the LIDC-IDRI dataset and preprocess data. The proposed CFBC algorithm is described in Sect. 3. In Sect. 4, a set of feature combination experiments are carried out and the properties of the considered operators are assessed using the classification result comparison method. The paper is concluded with a discussion in Sect. 5. Finally, conclusions are given in Sect. 6.

2 Data and Materials

LIDC-IDRI [21] is an open database in the cancer imaging archive (TCIA) for lung cancer diagnosis. It consists of 1010 clinical chest CT scans, each having an associated XML file that records not only location information of nodules on each slice but also nine characters, i.e. malignancy, texture, speculation, lobulation, margin, sphericity, calcification, internal structure, and subtlety. The appraisal value of each character is affected by up to four experienced thoracic radiologists. The malignancy rating of all nodules were evaluated from 1 to 5. Rating 1 denotes highly unlikely to be malignant, whereas rating 5 is highly suspicious. Please refer to [21] for more information about the database, such as the methods and protocols used in image acquisition.

We adopt the software tool in [22] to extract the lung nodule region and malignancy of a single 2D image slice. Once the lung nodule regions on all of the 2D slices were determined, the 3D volume of the nodule can be gained by superimposing all the 2D combination areas. We chose the diagnosis given by the only one experienced thoracic radiologist as the ground truth. Since the nodules with malignancy rating from 1 to 3 are regarded as benign and others as malignant, we have totally 1181 benign nodules and 387 malignant nodules.

3   CFBC Algorithm

The proposed CFBC nodule classification algorithm consists of four steps: (1) extracting DCNN features; (2) extracting texture and shape features; (3) using combined features to train a BP neural network as a slice-based classifier; and (4) classifying each lung nodule. The diagram of this algorithm is summarized in Fig. 1.

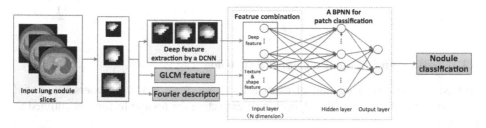

Fig. 1. Diagram of proposed CFBC nodule classification algorithm (Color figure online)

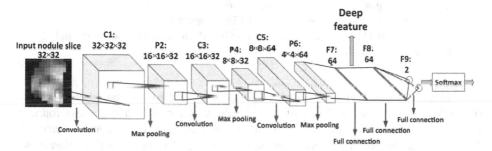

Fig. 2. Architecture of the DCNN in this study

3.1   DCNN-Based Feature Extraction

By identify a squared bounding box of lung nodules on a slice-by-slice basis, we obtain 9073 image patches from 1568 nodules. After resizing them into a dimension of 32×32 using the nearest interpolation algorithm, we apply these patches to train a nine-layer DCNN, which is constructed based on the LeNet-5 model [23].

As shown in Fig. 2, this DCNN consists of three convolution layers, three max-pooling layers and three full connected layers. Each convolution layer uses the ReLu activation function to implement a non-linear transformation from input to output. The parameters used in each layer are summarized in Table 1. In this study, we empirically set the learning rate to 0.001 and the maximum iteration number to 100, and chose the batch training style with the batch size of 100. As for other parameters, we adopted the default settings suggested in the MatConvNet Toolbox [24]. We define the output of the 7th layer of the trained network as the 64 dimensional DCNN feature extracted for the corresponding image patches.

Table 1. Parameter settings of each layer in the DCNN shown in Fig. 2

	C1	P2	C3	P4	C5	P6	F7	F8
Filter number	32	/	32	/	64	/	64	64
Filter size	5×5	/	5×5	/	5×5	/	5×5	1×1
Pooling size	/	3×3	/	3×3	/	3×3	/	/
Feature map	32×32	16×16	16×16	8×8	8×8	4×4	1×1	1×1
Pad	2	[0 1 0 1]	2	[0 1 0 1]	2	[0 1 0 1]	0	0
Stride	1	2	1	2	1	2	1	1

3.2   Texture and Shape Descriptor Extraction

GLCM is a statistical method of extracting texture feature and considers the spatial relationship of the pixels. The algorithm of extracting the texture features is outlined as follows.

Algorithm: GLCM texture descriptor calculation
1. Quantize the gray value of each pixel to 16 levels;
2. Count four GLCMs at $0°$, $45°$, $90°$ and $135°$, respectively;
3. Calculate four Haralick features on each GLCM on each direction separately for four directions in total.

Although Haralick et al. [25] defined fourteen textural features based on GLCM to quantify the spatial dependence of gray levels, it is recognized that those fourteen features are highly correlated and only the energy, contrast, entropy and inverse difference are irrelevant and effective enough for image classifications [26]. Hence, we calculated those four texture features on each GLCM and the calculation formulas can be found in paper [25]. Eventually, we obtained a 16-dimensional GLCM texture descriptor.

Fourier descriptor has an excellent performance in general shape analysis [11]. On each image patch, the Fourier descriptor is computed in four steps:

Algorithm: Fourier texture descriptor extraction
1. Identify the center of gravity on the binary image patch;
2. Move a point along the nodule counter and plot the distance between the point and gravity center versus the geodesic distance that the point moves;
3. Apply the Fourier transform to this plot.
4. Select 52 low frequency coefficients as the Fourier descriptor.

3.3   Patch Classification

Combing the DCNN feature, GLCM feature and Fourier descriptor, we have a 132-dimensional feature for each image patch. Then, we apply the combined features obtained on training samples to train a BP neural network, which contains one input layer with 132 neurons, one hidden layer with 132 neurons and one output layer with two neurons.

Since the DCNN model has already learned the best parameters, including the weights in the last three fully connected layers, we attempt to utilize those weights in the BP neural network [27] by dividing the BP weights into two groups. As shown in Fig. 1, the weights highlighted in red are directly copied from the DCNN and keep fixed, and only the weights in black will be adjusted during the training of the BP neural network. We set the maximum number of convergence to 50, learning rate to 0.001 and convergence error to 0.0004. As for other parameters, we adopted the default settings suggested in the BP neural network toolbox in Matlab. The trained BP neural network can predict the class label of each patch.

3.4   Nodule Classification

Each lung nodule appears on multiple slices. We first extract the DCNN feature, GLCM feature and Fourier descriptor with a squired bounding box on each slice. Then, we apply the combined feature to the trained BP neural network for label prediction. Finally, the class label of the nodule is determined by using majority voting based on the labels of it slices.

3.5   Evaluation

We evaluated the proposed CFBC nodule classification algorithm against those using one or two groups of features only. The LIDC-IDRI dataset consists of 1181 benign nodules and 387 malignant nodules. We evaluated the proposed nodule classification algorithm in four-fold cross validation. Each of the first three folds has 295 benign nodules and 97 malignant nodules for testing and others for training. The fourth fold has 296 benign nodules and 96 malignant nodules for testing and others for training. Such partition of the dataset ensures that each case will be tested once and only once. The nodule classification performance is assessed in terms of accuracy, sensitivity and specificity, which represent the rate of correctly classified cases, true positive rate and true negative rate, respectively [28].

4   Experimental Result

Table 2 gives the classification accuracy, sensitivity and specificity obtained by using DCNN features, GLCM features, Fourier shape descriptor alone or a combination of them. It shows that combining the DCNN features with either of the other two features can improve the classification accuracy, and the proposed algorithm that combines all three groups of features achieves the highest accuracy, sensitivity and specificity.

Table 2. Classification accuracy of different feature combinations

DCNN feature	GLCM feature	Fourier descriptor	BP neural network		
			Accuracy (%)	Sensitivity (%)	Specificity (%)
✓			82.92	53.85	92.21
	✓		83.65	47.44	95.42
		✓	83.02	53.85	92.50
	✓	✓	85.09	53.85	95.01
✓	✓		86.16	58.97	95.00
✓		✓	85.22	58.97	93.75
✓	✓	✓	**86.79**	**60.26**	**95.42**

Table 3 gives the performance of our algorithm and four state-of-the-art lung nodule classification approaches published in the literature. It reveals that our algorithm is substantially more accurate than other algorithms.

However, when compared to the method proposed by Hua [11], our method achieves higher specificity but lower sensitivity. It means that our method is more likely to diagnose a malignant nodule to be benign than Hua's method, and Hua's method is much more likely to diagnose a benign nodule to be malignant than our method. The poor sensitivity achieved by our method can be largely ascribed to its vulnerability to the unbalance in training data, i.e. 1181 benign versus 387 malignant nodules. In our future work, we will address this issue by adopting unbalance data analysis strategies used in traditional pattern classification, such as abandoning some data in the large group, resampling the small group and using penalty terms.

Table 3. Performance comparison of classification methods of lung nodules.

	Accuracy (%)	Sensitivity (%)	Specificity (%)
Arai et al. (2012) [29]	78.00	/	/
Hua et al. (2015) [20]	/	73.30	78.70
Kumar et al. (2015) [4]	75.01	83.35	/
Orozco et al. (2015) [30]	82	90.90	/
Our method	**86.79**	60.26	95.42

5   Discussion

It is straightforward to use a combination of different types of features to classify images. In our previous work, we have jointly used texture features and colour features for effective image classification and achieved relatively good results. However, when it comes to deep features, it seems not necessary to combine them with traditional visual features to attack large scale image classification problems, since deep models have already achieved remarkable success in these problems. However, when applied to medical image classification problems, where there usually is a small training dataset, deep models can hardly achieve a satisfying accuracy. The inaccuracy can be ascribed to the small training dataset, which leads deep models to over-fitting and cannot generate a representation that has the optimal discriminatory power. Therefore, we suggested that traditional visual features, particularly those extracted under the guidance of prior domain knowledge, may complement the features learned by deep models. Our experimental results demonstrate that this is true. In our next step, we will investigate if the performance improvement resulted from such feature combination becomes more significant when the training dataset gets even smaller.

Due to the use of DCNN, the proposed CFBC nodule classification algorithm has very high computation complexity during the off-line training. In our experiments, it costs us almost 24 h to train the proposed model (NVIDIA Tesla K40c GPU, 128 G RAM and Matlab 2012). However, applying the trained model to nodule classification is relatively fast, costing less than 0.5 s to classify each nodule on average. Therefore, we believe the proposed algorithm is applicable in clinical practices.

Another disadvantage of neural network-based approach is the involvement of a large number of parameters. Actually, tuning those parameters and the network structure remains an open problem, which becomes particularly difficult and time-consuming when the network gets deep. In this study, we adopted the suggested default settings for most of the parameters. Tuning those parameters will very likely further improve the performance of the proposed algorithm, but is obviously beyond the scope of this paper.

6 Conclusion

This paper proposes a novel CFBC nodule classification algorithm, which jointly uses the GLCM texture descriptor, Fourier shape descriptor and the features learned by a DCNN to differentiate malignant lung nodules from benign ones. Our experimental results on the benchmark LIDC-IDRI dataset suggest that combining the DCNN feature with traditional visual features can improve the accuracy of nodule classification and produce more accurate results than four state-of-the-art approaches. Our future work will focus on extending this slice-based approach to directly processing 3D data volumes.

Acknowledgement. This work was supported in part by the National Natural Science Foundation of China under Grants 61471297, in part by the Seed Foundation of Innovation and Creation for Graduate Students in Northwestern Polytechnical University under Grants Z2017041, and in part by the Australian Research Council (ARC) Grants. We acknowledge the National Cancer Institute and the Foundation for the National Institutes of Health, and their critical role in the creation of the free publicly available LIDC/IDRI Database used in this work.

References

1. Abraham, J.: Reduced lung-cancer mortality with low-dose computed tomographic screening. N. Engl. J. Med. **365**, 395–409 (2011)
2. Parkin, D.M.: Global cancer statistics in the year 2000. Lancet Oncol. **2**, 533–543 (2001)

3. Bach, P.B., Mirkin, J.N., Oliver, T.K., Azzoli, C.G., Berry, D., Brawley, O.W., Byers, T., Colditz, G.A., Gould, M.K., Jett, J.R.: Benefits and harms of CT screening for lung cancer: a systematic review. JAMA, J. Am. Med. Assoc. **307**, 2418–2429 (2012)

4. Kumar, D., Wong, A., Clausi, D.A.: Lung nodule classification using deep features in CT images. Comput. Robot Vis. **327**, 110–116 (2015)

5. Partio, M., Cramariuc, B., Gabbouj, M., Visa, A.: Rock texture retrieval using gray level co-occurrence matrix. In: Proceedings of the Nordic Signal Processing Symposium Norsig Norway (2002)

6. Wu, H., Sun, T., Wang, J., Li, X., Wang, W., Huo, D., Lv, P., He, W., Wang, K., Guo, X.: Combination of radiological and gray level co-occurrence matrix textural features used to distinguish solitary pulmonary nodules by computed tomography. J. Digit. Imaging **26**, 797–802 (2013)

7. Aggarwal, T., Furqan, A., Kalra, K.: Feature extraction and LDA based classification of lung nodules in chest CT scan images. In: 2015 International Conference on Advances in Computing, Communications and Informatics, pp. 1189–1193. IEEE Press, New York (2015)

8. Mabrouk, M., Karrar, A., Sharawy, A.: support vector machine based computer aided diagnosis system for large lung nodules classification. J. Med. Imaging Health Inform. **3**, 214–220 (2013)

9. Chang, C.C., Lin, C.J.: LIBSVM: a library for support vector machines. ACM Trans. Intell. Syst. Technol. **2**, 389–396 (2011)

10. Anand, S.K.V.: Segmentation coupled textural feature classification for lung tumor prediction. In: 2010 IEEE International Conference on Communication Control and Computing Technologies, pp. 518–524. IEEE Press, New York (2010)

11. Frejlichowski, D.: An experimental comparison of seven shape descriptors in the general shape analysis problem. In: Campilho, A., Kamel, M. (eds.) ICIAR 2010. LNCS, vol. 6111, pp. 294–305. Springer, Heidelberg (2010). doi:10.1007/978-3-642-13772-3_30

12. Sokic, E., Konjicija, S.: Shape description using phase-preserving Fourier descriptor. In: ICME 2015, pp. 1–6. IEEE Press, New York (2015)

13. Zhang, D., Lu, G.: Shape-based image retrieval using generic Fourier descriptor. Signal Process. Image **17**, 825–848 (2002)

14. Utkin, L.V., Chekh, A.I., Zhuk, Y.A.: Binary classification SVM-based algorithms with interval-valued training data using triangular and Epanechnikov kernels. Neural Netw. Off. J. Int. Neural Netw. Soc. **80**, 53–66 (2016)

15. Burges, C.J.C.: A tutorial on support vector machines for pattern recognition. Data Mining Knowl. Discov. **2**, 121–167 (1998)

16. Dandil, E., Cakiroglu, M., Eksi, Z., Ozkan, M.: Artificial neural network-based classification system for lung nodules on computed tomography scans. In: Soft Computing and Pattern Recognition, pp. 382–386 (2014)

17. Lee, S., Kouzani, A.Z., Hu, E.J.: Random forest based lung nodule classification aided by clustering. Comput. Med. Imaging Graph. Off. J. Comput. Med. Imaging Soc. **34**, 535–542 (2010)

18. Breiman, L.: Random forests. Mach. Learn. **45**, 5–32 (2001)

19. Hinton, G.E., Salakhutdinov, R.R.: Reducing the dimensionality of data with neural networks. Science **313**, 504–507 (2006)

20. Hua, K.L., Hsu, C.H., Hidayati, S.C., Cheng, W.H., Chen, Y.J.: Computer-aided classification of lung nodules on computed tomography images via deep learning technique. Oncotargets Ther **8**, 2015–2022 (2015)

21. Iii, S.G.A., Mclennan, G., Bidaut, L., Mcnittgray, M.F., Meyer, C.R., Reeves, A.P., Zhao, B., Aberle, D.R., Henschke, C.I., Hoffman, E.A.: The Lung Image Database Consortium (LIDC) and Image Database Resource Initiative (IDRI): a completed reference database of lung nodules on CT scans. Med. Phys. **38**, 915–931 (2011)
22. Lampert, T.A., Stumpf, A., Gançarski, P.: An empirical study into annotator agreement, ground truth estimation, and algorithm evaluation. IEEE Trans. Image Process. **25**(6), 2557–2572 (2016)
23. Lécun, Y., Bottou, L., Bengio, Y., Haffner, P.: Gradient-based learning applied to document recognition. Proc. IEEE **86**, 2278–2324 (1998)
24. Vedaldi, A., Lenc, K.: MatConvNet - convolutional neural networks for MATLAB. Eprint Arxiv (2014)
25. Haralick, R.M., Shanmugam, K., Dinstein, I.H.: Textural features for image classification. IEEE Trans. Syst. Man Cybern. **3**, 610–621 (1973)
26. Manivannan, K., Aggarwal, P., Devabhaktuni, V., Kumar, A., Nims, D., Bhattacharya, P.: Particulate matter characterization by gray level co-occurrence matrix based support vector machines. J. Hazard. Mater. **223–224**, 94–103 (2012)
27. Zipser, D., Andersen, R.A.: A back-propagation programmed network that simulates response properties of a subset of posterior. Nature **331**, 679–684 (1988)
28. Firmino, M., Angelo, G., Morais, H., Dantas, M.R., Valentim, R.: Computer-aided detection (CADe) and diagnosis (CADx) system for lung cancer with likelihood of malignancy. Biomed. Eng. Online **15**, 1–17 (2016)
29. Arai, K., Okumura, H., Herdiyeni, Y.: Comparison of 2D and 3D local binary pattern in lung cancer diagnosis. Int. J. Adv. Comput. Sci. Appl. **3**(4), 89–95 (2012)
30. Orozco, H.M., Villegas, O.O.V., Sánchez, V.G.C., Alfaro, M.D.J.N.: Automated system for lung nodules classification based on wavelet feature descriptor and support vector machine. Biomed. Eng. Online **14**, 1–20 (2015)

Representation Learning
for Cross-Modality Classification

Gijs van Tulder[1]([⊠]) and Marleen de Bruijne[1,2]

[1] Biomedical Imaging Group Rotterdam,
Erasmus MC University Medical Center, Rotterdam, The Netherlands
`g.vantulder@erasmusmc.nl`
[2] Image Group, Department of Computer Science,
University of Copenhagen, Copenhagen, Denmark

Abstract. Differences in scanning parameters or modalities can complicate image analysis based on supervised classification. This paper presents two representation learning approaches, based on autoencoders, that address this problem by learning representations that are similar across domains. Both approaches use, next to the data representation objective, a similarity objective to minimise the difference between representations of corresponding patches from each domain. We evaluated the methods in transfer learning experiments on multi-modal brain MRI data and on synthetic data. After transforming training and test data from different modalities to the common representations learned by our methods, we trained classifiers for each of pair of modalities. We found that adding the similarity term to the standard objective can produce representations that are more similar and can give a higher accuracy in these cross-modality classification experiments.

Keywords: Representation learning · Transfer learning · Autoencoders · Deep learning · Multi-modal image analysis

1 Introduction

Most classification techniques assume that they will be applied to data that comes from the same domain as the training data. In practice it may be necessary to use training data from a different domain. In medical image analysis, for example, it may happen that annotated training data is available but comes from a different scanner, or was made with different scanning protocols or different imaging modalities. Transfer learning methods handle these differences by transferring the knowledge learned in one domain and applying it to data from another domain. Some approaches do this by transforming the feature spaces, while others use instance weighting to give larger weights to training samples that look more similar to the target data (see [1] for a recent overview).

This paper proposes two representation learning approaches for transfer learning and applies those to a medical imaging problem. Representation learning [2] methods learn efficient, data-driven representations of the training data

© Springer International Publishing AG 2017
H. Müller et al. (Eds.): MCV/BAMBI 2016, LNCS 10081, pp. 126–136, 2017.
DOI: 10.1007/978-3-319-61188-4_12

and have shown good results in same-domain applications. We use these techniques to learn cross-domain representations that are not just efficient descriptions of the data, but are also similar across domains.

There is an obvious trade-off between learning a representation that provides efficient descriptions of data from one domain and learning a representation that is similar between domains. We discuss a hybrid learning objective that combines a standard representation learning objective, which tries to learn an efficient representation, with a similarity objective that minimises cross-domain differences. We use a weighted combination to find an optimal trade-off.

We suggest two models: a set of domain-specific autoencoders and an axial neural network. Both approaches learn a common representation, with a separate transformation for each domain. With autoencoders, this is achieved by training a separate autoencoder for each domain, whereas the axial neural network uses a single network that combines inputs from all domains. For both models, we include a similarity term in the learning objective to minimise the representation difference between corresponding samples from each domain.

Previous work on the combination of representation learning and transfer learning in medical image analysis can be separated in several groups. A popular approach is to transfer feature descriptors. These approaches reuse features that were learned from images from another domain, such as natural images or a different medical image dataset, and apply those to the target data with data-specific fine-tuning (e.g., [3,4]), but do not generally train cross-domain classifiers. Another group of approaches does train on data from different domains, but does so with a single feature transformation for all domains. Siamese networks [5], neural networks that are trained on data from different domains in parallel, fall in this category. These models are somewhat similar to the networks discussed in this paper, since both types of models are trained on paired samples. However, our methods learn a different transformation for each domain, which may work better if the domains are dissimilar.

We performed our experiments on data from the BRATS tumor segmentation challenge [6]. This multi-modal dataset contains brain scans made with four MRI sequences and manual annotations. In addition, we present experiments on a synthetic dataset derived from the BRATS images. Using the representations learned by our methods as the features, we measured the classification performance of random forest classifiers trained on data from one sequence and applied to another.

The rest of this paper is organised as follows. Section 2 describes our methods. The data and experiments are discussed in Sects. 3 and 4 and the results in Sect. 5. We end with a discussion and conclusion.

2   Methods

In order to learn the similarities between the different modalities, we assume that our dataset has corresponding samples from each modality. In practical terms: we apply our methods to registered scans of the same subjects scanned with each modality. This allows us to define learning objectives that minimise the representation difference between corresponding patches from each modality.

128   G. van Tulder and M. de Bruijne

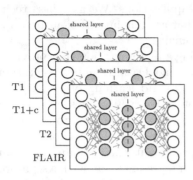

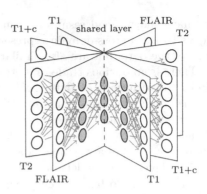

Fig. 1. We train a separate autoen-coder for each modality, with a sim-ilarity term that connects the central hidden layers across modalities.

Fig. 2. The axial neural network con-nects all modalities in a central axis, combining all inputs to get a common representation.

2.1 Autoencoders

Autoencoders [7] are multi-layer neural networks that consist of an input layer, a number of hidden layers and an output layer, with weighted directed connections between nodes in subsequent layers (Fig. 1). The input of the network is an image patch, with each node in the input layer representing one voxel. The first few hidden layers, the encoding part, compute an increasingly small representation of the input. The remaining layers form the decoding part and have an increasing number of nodes, up to the output layer that has the same number of nodes as the input. The network is trained to reconstruct the input, and because the number of nodes in the smallest hidden layer is limited, the model is forced to learn a concise representation of the data. This representation in the central hidden layer can be used as the feature vector for a classifier.

We used autoencoders with rectified linear units (ReLUs) [8] as the hidden nodes and nodes with a linear activation function for the final output layer. The connection weights of the encoding layers were shared by the decoding layers, but the biases of the encoding and decoding parts were independent.

For our experiments on multi-modal data, we trained a separate autoencoder for each of the M modalities. We have corresponding patches in each modality such that sample $\mathbf{x}_{m,i}$ contains the voxel values for patch i in modality m. We denote the values of the central hidden layer of the network for modality m given sample i by $f_m(\mathbf{x}_{m,i})$. Denote the values at the output layer by $g_m(f_m(\mathbf{x}_{m,i}))$. The network for modality m is trained to minimise the mean reconstruction error over all of the N training samples:

$$\mathcal{L}_{\mathrm{err},\,m} = \sum_{i=1}^{N} |g_m(f_m(\mathbf{x}_{m,i})) - \mathbf{x}_{m,i}|. \tag{1}$$

2.2   Learning Similar Representations

Training a separate autoencoder for each modality makes it possible to learn a different transformation for each modality, but does not learn a common representation across modalities. We extend the standard learning objective (1) with a similarity term that minimises the difference between the representation of a patch in one modality and its mean representation across modalities. We define the similarity objective for modality m as

$$\mathcal{L}_{\text{sim},\,m} = \sum_{i=1}^{N} \left| f_m\left(\mathbf{x}_{m,i}\right) - \frac{1}{M} \sum_{m'=1}^{M} f_{m'}\left(\mathbf{x}_{m',i}\right) \right|. \tag{2}$$

We combine this similarity objective with the standard autoencoder objective (1) to form a hybrid learning objective

$$\mathcal{L}_{\text{combined},\,m} = \alpha \mathcal{L}_{\text{sim},\,m} + (1 - \alpha)\, \mathcal{L}_{\text{err},\,m} \tag{3}$$

where the similarity weight α determines the trade-off between the representation error and the similarity objective. We vary this parameter in our experiments.

2.3   Axial Neural Networks

The axial neural network (Fig. 2) is a single model that combines all modalities. It has separate encoding layers for each modality, which are joined at a central hidden layer where the incoming representations are averaged into a single, shared representation. This shared representation is used as the input for the decoding part, which is again separate for each modality. For modality m, given the modality-specific encodings $f_{m'}$, the output is defined as

$$g_m\left(\frac{1}{M} \sum_{m'=1}^{M} f_{m'}\left(\mathbf{x}_{m',i}\right) \right). \tag{4}$$

Averaging over the representations encourages the model to learn a common representation that is similar across modalities. The network is trained using a learning objective that minimises the reconstruction error for each modality:

$$\mathcal{L}_{\text{err}} = \sum_{i=1}^{N} \sum_{m=1}^{M} \left| g_m\left(\frac{1}{M} \sum_{m'=1}^{M} f_{m'}\left(\mathbf{x}_{m',i}\right) \right) - \mathbf{x}_{m,i} \right|. \tag{5}$$

Similar to the approach with multiple autoencoders (3), the standard learning objective (5) can be combined with an additional similarity objective to explicitly minimise the differences between the representations coming from each modality:

$$\mathcal{L}_{\text{sim}} = \sum_{i=1}^{N} \sum_{m=1}^{M} \left| f_m\left(\mathbf{x}_{m,i}\right) - \frac{1}{M} \sum_{m'=1}^{M} f_{m'}\left(\mathbf{x}_{m',i}\right) \right| \quad \text{and} \tag{6}$$

$$\mathcal{L}_{\text{combined}} = \alpha \mathcal{L}_{\text{sim}} + (1 - \alpha)\, \mathcal{L}_{\text{err}}. \tag{7}$$

3   Data

We use data of 30 subjects from the BRATS tumor segmentation challenge [6] with four MRI sequences: T1, T1 post-contrast (T1+c), T2 and FLAIR (Fig. 3). The scans of each subject are rigidly registered to the T1+c scan and resampled to 1 mm isotropic resolution. The dataset contains brain masks and labels for four tumor components, some of which can only be identified on one specific sequence or by comparing multiple sequences [9]. Because our experiments require classes that can be identified on any single sequence, we grouped the four components in one foreground class and used the other parts of the brain mask as the background. For each subject we selected a balanced subset of 10 000 patches (11 × 11 × 5 voxels) for each class, taken at random positions inside the brain mask and at the same position for each sequence. We normalised each patch to zero mean and unit variance. We used the patches from 20 subjects for training, 5 subjects for validation of the random forest parameters and 5 for testing.

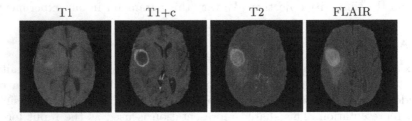

Fig. 3. One slice of the BRATS dataset shown in the four MRI sequences.

We also present experiments with an artifical dataset derived from the BRATS T1+c scans. Using four different MRI sequences makes it harder to see whether a low across-sequence performance is due to the different intensity distribution or simply because some structures are just not visible in one of the sequences. We therefore constructed an artificial dataset by transforming the T1+c scans with the exponential function $f(I) = I^\gamma$, where I is the voxel-wise intensity. Because each of the alternative views is derived from the same original scan, each view provides exactly the same information, but with a different distribution of intensity values. Before applying the transformation, we scaled the intensity values to fit between 0 and 1. We used the original intensities from the T1+c scan ($\gamma = 1$) and generated three alternative views computed with $\gamma = \{1.5, 2, 3\}$. After the transformation, each patch was normalised to zero mean and unit variance. We used the same set of training and test scans as in the other experiments.

4   Experiments

In our experiments we trained the autoencoders and axial neural networks on the patches in the BRATS dataset and the dataset with synthetic transformations.

For both scenarios, we trained the models to learn a joint representation for the four modalities. We evaluated multiple values for the weight of the similarity term in the learning objective. Using the learned representation as the feature vector, we then trained random forest classifiers and evaluated these by computing the classification accuracy on the test set. We did this for each pair of training and testing modalities.

We tried several network configurations for the autoencoders and axial neural networks. We used networks with three or five hidden layers, with 100 or 200 nodes in the central layer and 200 to 500 in the others. The number of nodes in the input and output layers was equal to the patch size, i.e., $11 \times 11 \times 5 = 605$ nodes. We trained networks for each combination of these parameters and used the performance on a held-out validation set to select the optimal combination.

As a baseline, we show the results of an approach that does not use different transformations for data from different modalities: we combined the patches from all modalities in one heterogeneous dataset and applied principal component analysis (PCA). We selected the 100 or 200 most important components, depending on the size of the network we compared with, to give the PCA baseline the same number of features as our models.

The networks were implemented in Python using Theano [10]. We trained the networks using stochastic gradient descent with a minibatch size of 50, for 300 epochs with various learning rates (0.0001, 0.001, 0.01 or 0.02). Based on our observations of the reconstruction and similarity objectives, we selected the networks with learning rates 0.001 and 0.01 for our classification experiments. We used the random forest implementation from Scikit-learn [11] for classification, with the number of trees (50, 75 or 100) optimised on the validation set.

5   Results

5.1   Synthetic Transformations

First, we present the results on the T1+c data with synthetic transformations. Figures 4 and 5 show the results averaged over the learning rates 0.02 and 0.01, which gave the best results on the training and validation sets. Choosing a similarity weight that is too large leads to suboptimal results, indicating that the networks learn uninformative representations if the similarity term is too strong and the reconstruction term too weak. For the smaller similarity weights, the patterns are different for the same-modality and different-modality scenarios. For same-modality training and test sets, learning representations that are similar across modalities is not important. For different-modality training and test data, the similarity term allows the models to learn similar representations for both datasets. Choosing the right weight for the similarity term brings the performance of different-modality training close to that of the same-modality baseline. This shows that the models learn representations that are similar across modalities.

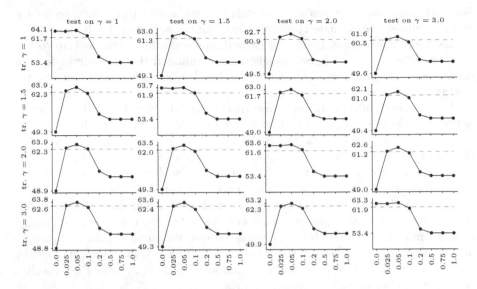

Fig. 4. Results with autoencoders and synthetic transformations of the T1+c scans. Classification accuracies (vertical axes) with features from autoencoders, for different modality pairs (rows and columns) and different weights of the similarity term (horizontal axes, 0 = no similarity). Dashed lines indicate the PCA result.

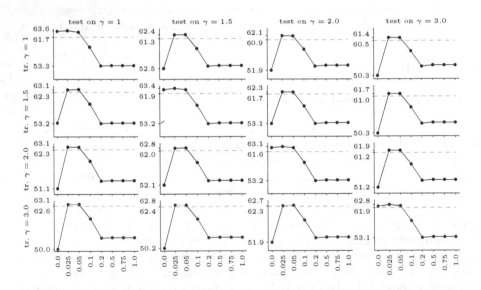

Fig. 5. Results with axial neural networks and synthetic transformations of the T1+c scans. Classification accuracies (vertical axes) with features from axial neural networks, for different modality pairs (rows and columns) and weights of the similarity term (horizontal axes, 0 = no similarity). Dashed lines indicate the PCA result.

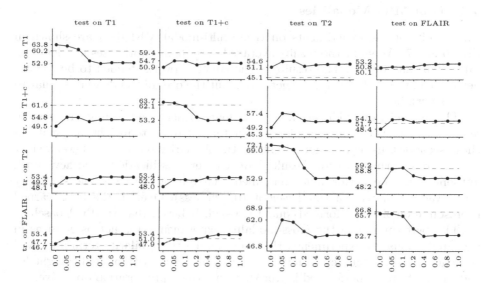

Fig. 6. Results with autoencoders and multi-modal BRATS data. Classification accuracies (vertical axes) with features from autoencoders, for different modality pairs (rows and columns) and different weights of the similarity term (horizontal axes, 0 = no similarity). Dashed lines indicate the PCA result.

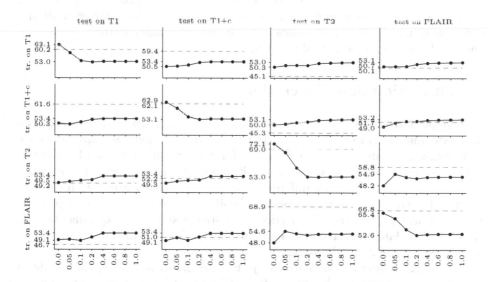

Fig. 7. Results with axial neural networks and multi-modal BRATS data. Classification accuracies (vertical axes) with features from axial neural networks, for different modality pairs (rows and columns) and weights of the similarity term (horizontal axes, 0 = no similarity). Dashed lines indicate the PCA result.

5.2   Four MRI Modalities

The results of the experiments on true multi-modal MRI data are shown in Figs. 6 and 7. We show the results averaged over the network sizes and learning rates (0.01 and 0.001). The results of the larger networks tended to be slightly better than those of the smaller networks, but the overall trends were similar to those shown here.

The best classification accuracy was found when the training and testing modalities were the same (the plots on the top-left to bottom-right diagonal). In these scenarios, using a larger weight for the similarity term and a lower weight for the reconstruction error resulted in a lower classification accuracy. With autoencoders, the performance remained relatively stable when the similarity term was added with a small weight (0.1 or less). Overall, the best learned representation often performed equal to or slightly better than the PCA baseline.

The performance in the cross-modality experiments was not as good as in the single-modality experiments. However, adding the similarity term improved the classification accuracy: a mixed learning objective with a small weight for the similarity term performed better than just the representation objective.

In scenarios with different training and testing modalities, the representations learned by our models usually gave a better classification accuracy than the representations made with PCA. PCA worked better for the pairings T1/T1+c and T2/FLAIR, perhaps because those sequences were more similar.

For the autoencoders, for certain modality pairs, the classification accuracy peaked at a similarity weight of 0.05 or 0.1, which corresponds to the plateau of the single-modality experiments. For other modality pairs, a larger similarity component gave a better classification accuracy. A similar pattern appears in the results for the axial neural networks.

6   Discussion and Conclusion

This paper introduced two representation learning approaches for learning similar representations from dissimilar data, using an additional learning objective that minimises representation differences for corresponding patches from different modalities. Our experiments on multi-modal MRI data showed that, when brain and test modalities are different, the representations learned with the similarity objective could produce better classification results than with just the normal learning objective. This effect was strongest in our experiments with simulated modalities derived from a single image, but was also visible in experiments on real multi-modal data.

Although adding the similarity objective can improve results, the weight of the objective should be chosen carefully. Giving a large weight to the similarity component favours learning a representation that is similar over learning a representation that is good at describing the data. This might cause the model to learn a trivial representation, such as all zeros, that may be similar across modalities but is not very useful for classification.

When training and testing on data from the same modality, adding the similarity objective may also lead to a lower performance, especially if the weight of the similarity objective is too large. For the autoencoders in our experiments, adding the similarity objective in a same-domain problem did not significantly decrease the accuracy if the weight of the similarity objective was small enough. This is useful when training a single model for use with multiple modalities.

While training and testing on different modalities may be less relevant in complete, multi-modal datasets such as BRATS, this scenario does have many practical applications. For example, approaches such as those proposed here allow data from different scanning protocols to be used for training a single model. The methods could also be used to suppress differences between scans made with scanners from different vendors. In multicenter studies it is possible to pool data from different modalities in a single model, avoiding the variability that may result from using separate models.

Cross-domain learning can only extract information that is visible in all domains and will have problems learning a common representation for structures visible in only one domain. The methods will therefore be most useful if the domains provide similar information but have different appearances. This is visible in the two sets of experiments in this paper. In the synthetic experiments, the modalities were all derived from the same post-contrast T1 image. This meant that each modality provided the same information – albeit with different intensity distributions – and the models could learn a shared representation that gave a good classification accuracy. In the experiments with real MRI modalities, on the other hand, performance depended on the modality pair. For example, post contrast T1 was analyzed best by models trained on that modality. T2 and the FLAIR appear to have more in common, but the cross-domain accuracy was still below the same-domain accuracy. This suggests that each modality provides additional information that is not available in the other modalities, which makes it harder to learn a shared representation.

We compared our methods with a fairly simple baseline, principal component analysis (PCA): by extracting the strongest variations in the data, PCA will likely extract common features that are shared between sources. PCA performed quite well for all modality pairs in our experiments on the synthetic dataset, which suggests that PCA is able to learn the artificial transformation that we applied there. This was not the case in our experiments on real multi-modal data, where the differences between the modalities are much more intricate. The power of PCA is limited because it has to use the same transformation for all modalities. This makes it impossible to learn, for instance, if the contrast of one of the modalities is inverted. In contrast, the methods proposed in this paper would be able to model these more complex transformations.

A conceptual advantage of axial neural networks is that they combine data from all domains in a single model, whereas autoencoders require an explicit similarity objective. However, in our experiments we found that autoencoders gave slightly better results, and that the performance of axial neural networks improved if we added an explicit similarity term.

Although the methods in this paper are unsupervised – the classifiers in our experiments were trained after the transformations had been learned – the general approach might also be applied with supervised methods, such as convolutional neural networks. In our axial neural network, for example, the decoding layers could be replaced by a set of output layers that compute class labels.

Using corresponding samples across domains is a powerful and efficient way to learn common representations, but it requires paired training samples. This data is available when, after introducing a new scanner, the same subject is scanned on the old and the new scanner. If there is no paired data, but there is labelled data from both domains, the class labels might provide a weaker form of correspondence between samples from the same class. Without class labels it may be possible to match the feature distribution of each domain.

In this paper we have shown two representation learning models that exploit sample correspondences to learn a common representation for samples from different domains. Using the common representation, a classifier can be trained on data from one domain and applied to data from another. Our experiments showed that classifiers trained on this common representation can, depending on the combination of modalities, achieve a higher accuracy than classifiers trained without the common representation.

References

1. Patel, V.M., Gopalan, R., Li, R., Chellappa, R.: Visual domain adaptation: a survey of recent advances. IEEE Signal Process. Mag. **32**, 53–69 (2015)
2. Bengio, Y., Courville, A., Vincent, P.: Representation learning: a review and new perspectives. Technical report, Université de Montréal (2012)
3. Shin, H.C., Roth, H.R., Gao, M., Lu, L., Xu, Z., Nogues, I., Yao, J., Mollura, D., Summers, R.M.: Deep convolutional neural networks for computer-aided detection: CNN architectures, dataset characteristics and transfer learning. IEEE Trans. Med. Imaging **35**, 1285–1298 (2016)
4. Tajbakhsh, N., Shin, J.Y., Gurudu, S.R., Hurst, R.T., Kendall, C.B., Gotway, M.B., Liang, J.: Convolutional neural networks for medical image analysis: fine tuning or full training? IEEE Trans. Med. Imaging **35**, 1299–1312 (2016)
5. Simo-Serra, E., Trulls, E., Ferraz, L., et al.: Discriminative learning of deep convolutional feature point descriptors. In: ICCV (2015)
6. Menze, B.H., Jakab, A., Bauer, S., et al.: The multimodal brain tumor image segmentation benchmark (BRATS). IEEE Trans. Med. Imaging **34**, 1993–2024 (2015)
7. Bengio, Y.: Learning deep architectures for AI. Found. Trends Mach. Learn. **2**(1), 1–127 (2009). http://www.nowpublishers.com/article/Details/MAL-006
8. Hinton, G.E.: A practical guide to training restricted Boltzmann machines. Technical report, University of Toronto (2010)
9. Jakab, A.: Segmenting brain tumors with the Slicer 3D software. Technical report, University of Debrecen (2012)
10. The Theano Development Team: Theano: a Python framework for fast computation of mathematical expressions. Technical report (2016)
11. Pedregosa, F., et al.: Scikit-learn: machine learning in Python. J. Mach. Learn. Res. **12**, 2825–2830 (2011)

Guideline-Based Machine Learning for Standard Plane Extraction in 3D Cardiac Ultrasound

Peifei Zhu[✉] and Zisheng Li

Hitachi, Ltd. Research and Development Group, Tokyo, Japan
{peifei.zhu.ww,zisheng.li.fj}@hitachi.com

Abstract. The extraction of six standard planes in 3D cardiac ultrasound plays an important role in clinical examination to analyze cardiac function. This paper proposes a guideline-based machine learning method for efficient and accurate standard plane extraction. A cardiac ultrasound guideline determines appropriate operation steps for clinical examinations. The idea of guideline-based machine learning is incorporating machine learning approaches into each stage of the guideline. First, Hough forest with hierarchical search is applied for 3D feature point detection. Second, initial planes are determined using anatomical regularities according to the guideline. Finally, a regression forest integrated with constraints of plane regularities is applied for refining each plane. The proposed method was evaluated on a 3D cardiac ultrasound dataset. Compared with other plane extraction methods, it demonstrated an improved accuracy with a significantly faster running time of 0.8 s per volume.

1 Introduction

3D cardiac ultrasound has become an increasingly common topic regarding imaging modalities. 3D ultrasound provides more cardiac information for evaluations compared with conventional 2D cardiac ultrasound. In a routine cardiac examination, clinicians usually use six standard planes, apical four chamber (A4C), apical two chamber (A2C), apical three chamber (A3C), parasternal short-axis mitral valve (PSX MV), parasternal short-axis papillary muscle (PSX PM), and parasternal short-axis apex (PSX AP) [1], to evaluate the structure and function of the heart. However, manual plane extraction suffers from inefficiency problems, such as user dependency and complex operational procedures. Therefore, an efficient and robust method for automatic plane extraction is extremely important in improving the cardiac examination workflow.

Previous works have proposed automatic extraction in 3D cardiac ultrasound volume. In [2], a database-driven knowledge-based approach is proposed for plane extraction. The method extracts image features from each standard plane and creates a probabilistic model [3]. During searching, a series of detectors are applied to estimate plane parameters, i.e., translation, orientation, and scale. False hypotheses at the earlier stages are removed, while right hypotheses are propagated to the final stage. However, large computational complexity for obtaining all plane parameters is still a problem, and the correct plane might also be missed at an earlier stage during search. In [4], the

© Springer International Publishing AG 2017
H. Müller et al. (Eds.): MCV/BAMBI 2016, LNCS 10081, pp. 137–147, 2017.
DOI: 10.1007/978-3-319-61188-4_13

locations of planes are considered as continuous parameters, and a regression voting approach is used to solve it. Regression forest [5] incorporated with voxel class information is used to train classifiers. During testing, every voxel of the cardiac volume provides votes on the parameters of each plane. The votes from all voxels are collected to produce a probability distribution, and the location of the plane is determined by the parameter with maximum probability. However, each plane is extracted independently in this approach, which means each voxel of the volume should pass through the classifier repeatedly (six times for six standard planes). This causes large computational complexity and is time consuming. In addition, anatomical regularities of standard planes, i.e., three apical planes should pass through the same center axis (apical long axis) [1], were not considered in [4]. Such knowledge is important in diagnosis and should also be incorporated into the process of plane extraction.

This paper proposes a new machine learning framework based on the cardiac ultrasound guideline (presented by the American Society of Echocardiography [1]) for standard plane extraction. The guideline has been established for clinicians to learn appropriate operation procedures for high quality cardiac examination. The proposed method is completely based on the guideline. Each stage in the guideline is achieved

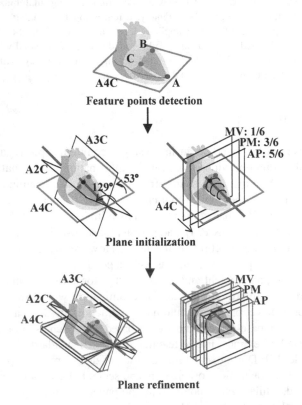

Fig. 1. Framework of guideline-based machine learning for standard plane extraction.

using an appropriate machine learning approach that yields guideline-based machine learning. The framework of the proposed method is shown in Fig. 1, and the process is as follows.

1. [Feature point detection] The guideline indicates searching the A4C plane using mitral annulus and apical features. Three anatomical feature points are selected correspondingly, and a Hough forest classifier [6, 7] with a hierarchical search is applied for detecting these points.
2. [Plane Initialization] The guideline indicates the anatomical regularities between A4C and the other five planes. Correspondingly, the initial locations of the other five planes are determined using these regularities.
3. [Plane refinement] Refinement is needed considering individual differences around the initial location. A regression forest method with locations constraints is applied for plane refinement.

This work makes three main contributions. First, it presents guideline-based machine learning that incorporates machine learning approaches into each stage of the guideline. This can also be applied to various measurements in medical images. Second, it presents a method using a Hough forest with hierarchical search for efficiently and accurately detecting 3D feature points. Third, location constraints are integrated into the regression forest for plane refinement, further improving the accuracy of plane extraction.

2 Standard Plane Initialization

According to the guideline, the A4C plane is first extracted by using mitral annulus and apical features. In the proposed method, three anatomical feature points, including the apex, left mitral annulus (left MA), and right mitral annulus (right MA), are selected correspondingly to localized plane A4C. Feature point detection is achieved using a Hough forest classifier, which is presented in Sect. 2.1. Moreover, a hierarchical search, presented in Sect. 2.2, is applied for improving the accuracy and speed. Then, as presented in Sect. 2.3, the initial locations of the six planes can be determined using the detected points and anatomical regularities all at once.

2.1 Hough Forest

Hough forest is used for detecting feature points. This method provides a way to map from image patches to anatomical locations. In this work, Hough forest is extended for 3D point detection using 3D image features and 3D Hough voting.

Training process: Each tree T of Hough forest is constructed based on a set of patches $\{P_i = (\mathbf{I_i}, c_i, \mathbf{d_i})\}$, where $\mathbf{I_i}$ is the appearance of the 3D patch, c_i is the class label that includes the positive class and negative class, and $\mathbf{d_i}$ is the offset from the patch center to the object center. The proportion between object patches and background patches C_L and the list $\mathbf{D_L} = \{\mathbf{d_i}\}$ of the offset vectors are stored for each leaf node L. Hough forest classifier is constructed from the root using the input patches. A key point of Hough forest is the evaluation of the binary test. To conduct an optimal test, the uncertainties in both the class labels and the offset vectors should decrease towards the leaves. A set of patches is defined as A= $\{P_i = (I_i, c_i, \mathbf{d_i})\}$, and class label uncertainty $U_1(A)$ and offset uncertainty $U_2(A)$ are defined as:

$$U_1(A) = -|A| \cdot \sum p(c|A) \ln(p(c|A)), \tag{1}$$

$$U_2(A) = \sum_i (\mathbf{d_i} - \mathbf{d_A})^2, \quad when\ c_i = 1, \tag{2}$$

where $|A|$ is the number of patches, $p(c|A)$ is the proportion of patches with label c in set A, and $\mathbf{d_A}$ is the mean offset vector over all object patches. Given a training set of patches, a pool of pixel tests $\{t_k\}$ is generated by randomly choosing one feature channel and two pixel locations inside a patch. The randomized decision is made as to whether the node should minimize the class-label uncertainty or the offset uncertainty. The process can be represented as:

$$\arg\min(U_*(\{P_i|t^k(\mathbf{I_i}) = 0\}) + U_*(\{P_i|t^k(\mathbf{I_i}) = 1\})), \tag{3}$$

where * is either the class label uncertainty or offset uncertainty.

Testing process: Testing can be considered as regression and voting steps. The regression process is as follows. (1) For each voxel location $\mathbf{p}$, a patch is extracted and starts regression from the root; (2) when passing each node, this patch is sorted into the left or right child node in accordance with the binary test. All pixels in the image go through the forest until they reach the leaves. During the voting process, the information stored in leaves is used to cast the probabilistic Hough votes to the location of the object center. The leaf information consists of proportion C_L and offset vectors $\mathbf{D_L}$, so $C_L/\mathbf{D_L}$ is defined as a weight value for a vote. Each pixel in leaves carries a location $\mathbf{p}$, and it votes to all locations $\{\mathbf{p} - \mathbf{d}|\mathbf{d} \in \mathbf{D_L}\}$ with a weight value $C_L/\mathbf{D_L}$. After all votes from each voxel have been summed up, the 3D Hough image can be obtained. Finally, the feature points are the locations with the maximum number of votes.

2.2   Hough Forest with Hierarchical Search

In Hough forest, the whole image is used during the testing step to cast the probabilistic Hough votes to the location of the object. When dealing with volume data, the regression of a huge number of 3D patches through forest will cause massive computations. In this work, a coarse-to-fine strategy is applied to accelerate the detection process. Feature points are detected serially through a multi-scale hierarchical search.

In the coarse-to-fine strategy, the whole image is first used to provide an estimate of the region of interest, which is then refined by using only local information. The framework is shown in Fig. 2. A coarse-level classifier and a fine-level classifier need to be trained before testing. The coarse classifier is trained using low-resolution images that are down-sampled from original images. Positive patches are chosen from a bounding box region around ground-truth, and negative patches are chosen from the whole image except the positive region. The fine-level classifier is trained on a high-resolution image (original image) with a sampling region narrowed down. During the testing step, first, the input image is down-sampled, and a coarse position is localized using Hough forest coarse-level classifier. In coarse-level detection, every pixel in a low-resolution image provides a vote (Hough voting) to a potential target location. Second, in the refinement step, only pixels in the neighborhood of the coarse position are used to predict the existence of the object. By applying a coarse-to-fine strategy, the searching region has largely been cut down, so the running time is successfully shortened. Moreover, refinement searching that only uses the region closest to the target can reduce the irrelevant information and provide higher accuracy.

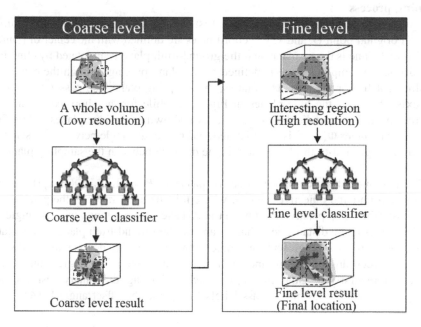

Fig. 2. Coarse-to-fine strategy applied for the Hough forest classifier.

2.3 Plane Initialization Using Anatomical Regularity

The initial locations of six standard planes can be determined using three feature points and the anatomical regularity defined in [1], shown in Fig. 1. First, the A4C plane passes through three feature points. The long-axis can also be localized by A and the center of B and C. A3C and A2C are intersected with the A4C plane at angles of approximately 53 ° and 129 °, respectively. Three short-axis planes (PSX MV, PM, and AP) are perpendicular to A4C and can be localized by translating along the long-axis with proportional intervals of 1/6, 3/6, and 5/6, respectively.

3   Regression Forest for Plane Refinement

The average anatomical regularities defined in [1] are estimated. Because the plane location has individual differences, each plane around the initial location needs refinement. This work proposes a method that incorporates location constraints into regression forest for plane refinement. The refinement can be categorized into two types according to the location constraints: (1) three long-axis planes (A4C, A3C, and A2C) should pass through the long-axis; (2) three short-axis planes (MV, PM, and AP) should be perpendicular to the long-axis. Correspondingly, either angle or distance of the initial plane will be refined, as shown in Fig. 3. To reduce the inference of irrelevant image information, background and object regions are also set in regression forest, similar to Hough forest.

Training process
Some important planes and parameters are first defined. The center of the 3D volume is set as an original point O, and x, y, z coordinates are defined with the center of point O. The original plane is the xz plane, and the ground-truth plane is annotated by clinicians. In addition, the sampling plane is defined as the plane passing through the center of a sampling patch. For the long-axis planes, the sampling plane also passes through the long-axis, shown as the blue planes in Fig. 3(a), while for the short-axis planes, the sampling plane is perpendicular to the long-axis, shown as the blue planes in Fig. 3(b). An offset parameter $\Phi(\theta, \gamma)$ is then defined, where θ is the angle between the sampling plane and the ground-truth plane, and γ is the distance between the sampling plane and the ground-truth plane.

The training dataset comprises a set of patches $\{P_i = (\mathbf{I_i}, c_i, \Phi(\theta, \gamma))\}$ sampled from background and objective regions, where $\mathbf{I_i}$ is the appearance of the patch, and c_i is the class label. The positive training set is collected from a range with an angle less than θ_τ degrees and a distance less than γ_τ around the ground-truth plane. The negative training set is from a range with an angle between $\theta_\tau \sim 2\theta_\tau$ degrees and a distance $\gamma_\tau \sim 2\gamma_\tau$ between around the ground-truth plane. Each tree of the regression forest is constructed recursively using the input patches. During the binary test for node training, the uncertainties in the class labels $V_1(A)$ and the offset angle $V_2(A)$

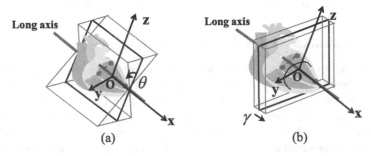

(a)   (b)

Fig. 3. Examples of standard plane refinement. (a) Angle refinement is applied for three long-axis planes. (b) Distance refinement is applied for three short-axis planes.

are defined as:

$$V_1(A) = -|A| \cdot \sum p(c|A),$$ (4)

$$V_2(A) = \sum_i (\Phi_i - \Phi_A)^2, \quad when \ c_i = 1,$$ (5)

where Φ_A is the mean offset parameter over all sampled patches. For obtaining an optimal test, the node should minimize the class-label uncertainty or the offset parameter uncertainty, which can be represented as

$$\arg\min(V_*(\{P_i | t^k(\mathbf{I_i}) = 0\}) + V_*(\{P_i | t^k(\mathbf{I_i}) = 1\})),$$ (6)

where $*$ is either class label uncertainty or offset uncertainty. Finally, for each leaf node, the proportion of the object patches and the background patches C_L, and the list $\{\Phi_i\}$ of the offset angle are stored.

Testing process.
The refinement regions are first defined. For the long-axis planes, the refinement region is set as an angle of $(-2\theta_\tau, 2\theta_\tau)$ around the initial planes, shown in Fig. 3(a). For the short-axis planes, the refinement region is set as a distance of $(-2\gamma_\tau, 2\gamma_\tau)$ centered at the initial planes, as shown in Fig. 3(b). Given a new unseen volume, all voxels of the refinement regions are pushed through each tree of forest until they reach leaf nodes. Leaf information consists of the proportion C_L, and the offset parameter $\{\Phi_i\}$. The proportion can be used for determining a threshold τ to control the minimum presence of the class label at each leaf and for use as a probability for the votes this leaf generates.

The voxel then votes for the location of the target plane $\Phi_t(\theta_t, \gamma_t)$ using the proportion C_L and the offset parameter $\{\Phi_i\}$ stored in the leaf. The process is as follows. First, the plane passing through the sampling voxel and the long-axis is calculated. $\Phi_p(\theta_p, \gamma_p)$ is marked as the angle and distance difference between this plane and the original plane. Therefore, a vote on the location of the target plane $\Phi_t = \Phi_p - \Phi_i$ is generated. All votes generated by the voxels can be summed up, and the final angle of the plane can be determined by the mean value $\overline{\Phi_t} = \sum_{L \in F} \Phi_t \cdot C_L / N$, where $L \in F$ means all leaves in the forest, and N is the total number of votes. Finally, the target plane can determine the original plane and the voted parameter $\overline{\Phi_t}$.

4 Experiments

The proposed method was evaluated on a 3D cardiac ultrasound dataset that was available in [8]. The dataset included cardiac cycle volumes from 15 volunteers. Volume dimensions were around $320 \times 347 \times 241$ with a resolution of $0.5 \ mm^3$. The end diastole frame from each of the volunteers was used. A 5-fold cross-validation scheme was applied for the evaluation. In addition, a data augmentation scheme was also applied with artificially rotating and scaling of the original volume. Therefore, 120 volumes were used for training, and 30 volumes were used for testing in each validation.

4.1   Evaluation of Feature Point Detection

The performance of the feature point detection was first evaluated. The point detection was conducted using two methods to compare the performance: (1) Hough forest and (2) Hough forest with hierarchical search (proposed method). The following parameter settings were used for all the classifiers: maximum tree depth $D = 15$, number of trees $T = 10$, and the threshold for separating the objective leaf and background leaf was $\tau = 0.95$. In addition, the image features used in this work include intensity, difference, and gradient features.

Distance error was used as a standard for the evaluation. Ground-truth points were annotated by a clinical expert manually. The distance error is the Euclidean distance between the ground-truth and the detected points. The comparison results of two methods are shown in Table 1. The distance error of each of the feature points and the mean distance error of all three points were calculated, and they are shown in mean ± standard deviation format. The comparison results demonstrated that the proposed method reduced the mean distance error of the three points by about 23.6% and also improved the speed by about 10 times. The improvement in the accuracy and speed was attributed to a coarse-to-fine strategy. The searching region was largely reduced, enabling a significantly shorter running time. Moreover, only regions that were close to the target were used. This reduced the irrelevant information and provided higher accuracy. Examples of detection images by Hough forest, the proposed method, and a ground-truth image are shown in Fig. 4. The images are the A4C plane localized using three feature points. The proposed method showed improved accuracy for all of the feature points.

Table 1. Comparison of point detection between Hough forest and proposed method.

	Distance error (mm)				Run time (s)
	Apex	Left MA	Right MA	Mean	–
Hough forest [6]	12.2 ± 4.3	8.1 ± 3.9	6.5 ± 3.8	8.9 ± 4.0	4.5
Proposed method	**10.5 ± 4.2**	**4.9 ± 3.5**	**5.1 ± 3.3**	**6.8 ± 3.7**	**0.45**

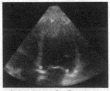 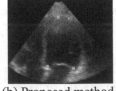 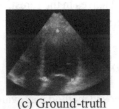

(a) Hough forest   (b) Proposed method   (c) Ground-truth

Fig. 4. Examples of feature point detection by Hough forest and proposed method. Ground-truth has manually annotated points for comparison.

4.2 Evaluation of Plane Extraction

Two evaluation standards were introduced, angle error and distance error, to measure the difference between the ground-truth plane and the extracted plane [2]. The angle error between two planes was defined as the angle between the normal vector of the ground-truth plane and the normal vector of the extracted plane. The distance error between two planes was measured as the distance from an anchor on one plane to the other plane, where the anchor was the LV center. The ground-truth planes were all annotated by clinical experts manually. During the manual annotation, the standard planes were determined by image features and anatomical regularities. For example, the PSX MV plane is at the base cardiac left ventricle, and a common feature of this plane is the so-called "goldfish mouth" look of the mitral valve leaflets.

Comparison results between applying the refinement before and after are shown in Table 2. Six standard planes were categorized into two types. The long-axis planes include A4C, A3C, and A2C, and the short-axis planes include PSX MV, PSX PM, and PSX AP. The mean angle error and distance error of both types were calculated. The results show that improved accuracy was achieved after refinement. The mean angle error of the long-axis planes and mean distance error of short-axis planes were reduced by about 16.9% and 46.9%, respectively. The results demonstrate the effectiveness of the angle and distance refinement using the proposed method. Examples of standard plane extraction are shown in Fig. 5. The extraction results before refinement, after refinement, and the ground-truth were compared. Using the refinement obviously improved detailed information such as the region near the aortic valve on plane A3C.

In another experiment, the performance of the proposed method was compared to that of other plane extraction methods. The results are shown in Table 3. The average angle and the distance error of all six planes were calculated. All kinds of error are shown in mean ± standard deviation format. The running time was all measured as the total extracting time of six planes, and all the experiments were run on an Intel core i7 3.6 GHz computer with 16 GB of RAM. The proposed method was compared with marginal space learning (MSL) [2] and class-specific regression forest (RF) [4], which were all introduced in Sect. 1. As shown in Table 3, the angle and distance error of the proposed method was reduced by about 30% compared with those of MSL, while the running time of the proposed method was significantly shorter than that of the class-specific RF.

Table 2. Comparison results of standard plane extraction between applying the refinement before and after.

	Three long-axis planes		Three short-axis planes	
	Angle (degrees)	Distance (mm)	Angle (degrees)	Distance (mm)
Before refinement	11.8 ± 6.2	2.8 ± 2.5	6.9 ± 4.0	4.9 ± 3.1
After refinement	9.8 ± 5.8	2.8 ± 2.3	6.8 ± 4.0	2.6 ± 2.3

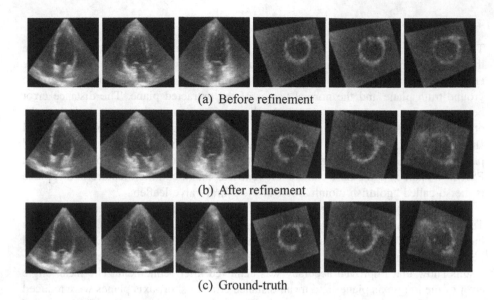

(a) Before refinement

(b) After refinement

(c) Ground-truth

Fig. 5. Examples of standard plane extraction. The six planes from left to right are: A4C, A3C, A2C, PSX AP, PSX PM, and PSX MV. From top to bottom: (a) Before refinement: initialization planes determined by feature points and anatomical regularity. (b) After refinement: planes with a refinement around the initial location. (c) Ground-truth: manually annotated planes.

Table 3. Comparison results of standard plane extraction between proposed method and other plane extraction methods.

	Angle (degrees)	Distance (mm)	Run time (s)
MSL [2]	11.3 ± 8.0	3.7 ± 2.1	2
Class-specific RF [4]	6.4 ± 4.3	4.2 ± 3.8	30
Proposed method	**8.3 ± 4.9**	**2.7 ± 2.3**	**0.8**

4.3   Discussion

The following factors can be attributed to the improved performance: (1) the proposed method is based on the guideline, where the anatomical regularities are incorporated into determining the initial plane locations. The search regions of each plane were largely cut down. (2) In feature point detection, a coarse-to-fine strategy is proposed for Hough forest classifier, and it also reduces the search region and cuts down noises. (3) The refinement around the initial location using regression forest further improves the extraction accuracy. The proposed method can be further accelerated by using parallel processing on both Hough forest and regression forest. However, the problems remained in the work are the small number of the evaluation data and the lack of the inter-observer variability. In the future, more data will be collected for evaluation. Moreover, more than two experts will be asked to annotate the standard planes from same image to improve the inter-observer variability.

5 Conclusions

This paper proposed a new machine learning framework based on the cardiac ultrasound guideline for standard-plane extraction. Each stage in the guideline is achieved using an appropriate machine learning approach. Hough forest with hierarchical search was proposed for detecting efficient and robust feature points. After six planes are extracted by anatomical regularity, a refinement step using regression forest is applied to improve the accuracy further. Experimental results demonstrated that the proposed method improved performance in both accuracy and speed compared with other methods.

References

1. Lang, R.M., Badano, L.P., et al.: Recommendations for cardiac chamber quantification by echocardiography in adults: an update from the American Society of Echocardiography and the European Association of Cardiovascular Imaging. J. Am. Soc. Echocardiogr. **28**(1), 1–39 (2015)
2. Lu, X., Georgescu, B., et al.: Automated detection of planes from three-dimensional echocardiographic data. U.S. Patent No. 8,073,215. 6, December 2011
3. Zheng, Y., Barbu, A., et al.: Fast automatic heart chamber segmentation from 3D CT data using marginal space learning and steerable features. In: International Conference on Computer Vision (ICCV) (2007)
4. Chykeyuk, K., Yaqub, M., Alison Noble, J.: Class-specific regression random forest for accurate extraction of standard planes from 3D echocardiography. In: Menze, B., Langs, G., Montillo, A., Kelm, M., Müller, H., Tu, Z. (eds.) MCV 2013. LNCS, vol. 8331, pp. 53–62. Springer, Cham (2014). doi:10.1007/978-3-319-05530-5_6
5. Criminisi, A., Shotton, J., Robertson, D., Konukoglu, E.: Regression forests for efficient anatomy detection and localization in CT studies. In: Menze, B., Langs, G., Tu, Z., Criminisi, A. (eds.) MCV 2010. LNCS, vol. 6533, pp. 106–117. Springer, Heidelberg (2011). doi:10.1007/978-3-642-18421-5_11
6. Gall J, Lempitsky V.: Class-specific Hough forests for object detection. In: Decision forests for Computer Vision and Medical Image Analysis, pp. 143–157. Springer, London (2013)
7. Gall, J., Yao, A., Razavi, N., et al.: Hough forests for object detection, tracking, and action recognition. IEEE Trans. Pattern Anal. Mach. Intell. **33**(11), 2188–2202 (2011)
8. Tobon-Gomez, C., De Craene, M., et al.: Benchmarking framework for myocardial tracking and deformation algorithms: An open access database. Med. Image Anal. **17**(6), 632–648 (2013)

BAMBI Workshop

A Statistical Model for Simultaneous Template Estimation, Bias Correction, and Registration of 3D Brain Images

Akshay Pai[1,2]($\boxtimes$), Stefan Sommer[1], Lars Lau Raket[3], Line Kühnel[1],
Sune Darkner[1], Lauge Sørensen[1,2], and Mads Nielsen[1,2]

[1] DIKU, University of Copenhagen, Copenhagen, Denmark
[2] Biomediq A/S, Copenhagen, Denmark
akshay@biomediq.com
[3] Lundbeck, Copenhagen, Denmark

Abstract. Template estimation plays a crucial role in computational anatomy since it provides reference frames for performing statistical analysis of the underlying anatomical population variability. While building models for template estimation, variability in sites and image acquisition protocols need to be accounted for. To account for such variability, we propose a generative template estimation model that makes simultaneous inference of both bias fields in individual images, deformations for image registration, and variance hyperparameters. In contrast, existing maximum a posterori based methods need to rely on either bias-invariant similarity measures or robust image normalization. Results on synthetic and real brain MRI images demonstrate the capability of the model to capture heterogeneity in intensities and provide a reliable template estimation from registration.

1 Introduction

Brain template estimation is becoming increasingly important since it facilitates a variety of applications such as segmentation, registration, or providing common coordinate systems for statistical analysis of shape models for a given population. At the core of template estimation methods is image registration. In a statistical setting, conventional image registration methods are often approached from a Bayesian viewpoint where one maximizes the posterior given the image data and a regularizing prior [1]. To avoid choosing parameters for controlling the deformation (regularization) in an ad-hoc fashion, recent methods have employed Bayesian models where parameters are estimated in a data-driven fashion by treating them as latent random variables drawn from a distribution with a smooth covariance structure [2,3]. These methods employ L^2 similarity measures that are fragile towards deviations in model assumption; for instance, bias fields. To achieve reasonable results under model deviations, strong penalization on the variation in deformation parameters can be imposed, or similarity measures that are invariant to bias fields (e.g. mutual information) can be used instead of the L^2 data terms.

H. Müller et al. (Eds.): MCV/BAMBI 2016, LNCS 10081, pp. 151–159, 2017.
DOI: 10.1007/978-3-319-61188-4_14

In this paper, we propose a statistical mixed-effects model where deformation and spatially correlated variation in intensity are modeled as random effects. This way, effects from deformations and variations in intensities due to scanners can be separately handled, and hyperparameters can be estimated in a data-driven fashion using maximum likelihood. We perform simultaneous estimation and prediction in the model to avoid bias in the estimation that can result from treating warping as a preprocessing step [4]. In addition, we propose a different estimation procedure in comparison to existing Bayesian methods. While current methods use non-linear sampling for marginalizing over the latent variables, we propose to use successive linearization around predictions of the latent variables allowing estimation with linear mixed-effect theory. This paper is built on the methods proposed by Raket et al. [4] for analysis of 1D functional data.

Current probabilistic template estimation methods do not model multi-scale behavior of the deformations. Although innumerable multi-scale deformation models have been proposed for image registration, their application in template estimation still needs maturity. To this end, we propose to model deformations at different scales as latent variables that are drawn from different distributions with different covariance structure. Concretely, we utilize the kernel bundle structure [5,6] to model velocity fields, and the multi-scale nature is interleaved in the covariance structure of the distribution of parameters at each kernel bundle level.

The contributions of the paper are as follows:

- We demonstrate the utility of a computationally feasible class of non-linear mixed effect models in 3D brain template estimation.
- We propose a model that handles effects from deformation and intensity variations separately and allows simultaneous estimation of template and variance hyperparameters and prediction of deformation and bias fields.
- We propose an iterative linearization of the model in the non-linear random effects that enables efficient maximum likelihood estimation of variance parameters.
- Finally, we propose the incorporation of scales in the deformation distribution via the kernel bundle representation.

2   Background

A number of registration-based approaches to template estimation have been proposed where the central aspect addressed was the choice of target co-ordinate system. Initial approaches, which include the popular minimum deformation template [7], choose a random image as a target co-ordinate system, and is iteratively updated by registering other images to it. This approach has been shown to be significantly biased towards the choice of the random image [8].

As an alternate approach, several papers have proposed the strategy of registering several images to a template, which is simultaneously estimated via an alternating optimization scheme [9,10]. In a probabilistic formulation, the image matching term can be viewed as a log likelihood and the regularization as a log prior. In this direction, recent methods like [3] have employed tools such as non-linear mixed effects models to deal with the population effects (template or the fixed effect) and individual effects (deformations or the random effect). Methods have moved towards simultaneously modeling the template and inferring parameters of the deformation such as the regularization factor with expectation-maximization [2]. All the aforementioned methods rely on bias-invariant similarity measures or robust image normalization methods. To address intensity bias factors, Hromatka et al. [11], proposed to use a hierarchical Bayesian model for template estimation where two transformations are concatenated; one taking an individual image to an atlas of a site and the other that takes this warped image to the global atlas. However, this model takes into consideration very little about intra-site bias variations.

3   Statistical Model

Consider a population of images $I_i : \mathbb{R}^3 \to \mathbb{R}, i = 1 \ldots k$ and let θ be a template of these images; both measured on a discrete grid $\Omega \in \mathbb{Z}^3$. The individual observed image may be then defined in terms of the fixed and random effects as

$$I_i = \theta(\text{Exp}(v(w_i)) + x_i + \epsilon_i \tag{1}$$

where the template θ is the fixed effect. More control over the smoothness of θ may be incorporated by specifying a parametric subspace for θ. However, such constructions will not be entertained in this paper. The remaining effects are all random: The deformation $\text{Exp}(v(w_i))$ (Sect. 3.2) is a random field controlled by latent random deformation parameters w_i. A key contribution of this paper is the incorporation of the random spatially correlated effect x_i that models a bias field. Note that x_i is defined in the frame of the individual image and not the template. Converse constructions are also possible. Finally, ϵ_i is the i.i.d noise.

Following [4] and assuming that θ is smooth, we can linearize (1) around deformation parameters w_i^0 resulting in the linear model

$I_i \approx \theta^{w_i^0} + Z_i(w_i - w_i^0) + x_i + \epsilon_i$, where,

$\theta^{w_i^0} = \theta(\text{Exp}(v(w_i^0)))$, $Z_i = \nabla_{\mathbf{x}}\theta(\text{Exp}(v(w_i^0)))^T|_{\mathbf{x}=\text{Exp}(v(w_i^0))} J_w \text{Exp}(v(w_i^0)) \in \mathbb{R}^{n \times n_w}$,

$w_i \sim \mathcal{N}(0, \sigma^2 C_i)$, $C_i = \mathbb{I}_i \otimes C_0$, $x_i \sim \mathcal{N}(0, \sigma^2 S_i)$, $S_i = \mathbb{I}_i \otimes S_0$,

$\epsilon_i \sim \mathcal{N}(0, \sigma^2 \mathbb{I}_i)$.

Here σ^2 is the noise variance, and the spatial covariance of the deformations and bias fields are controlled by the matrices C and S. Note that $\nabla_{\mathbf{x}}$ denotes derivatives with respect to spatial coordinates. Also, note that deformations in the linear model are parameters of w while the linearization point w^0 is iteratively optimized for during the estimation process. The model here is a single scale model where the covariances are constructed with only one scale of the kernel. Multi-scale version of this will be discussed in Sect. 3.2.

The first step of the analysis is to estimate θ with an initial guess of linearization point w. θ is computed by back-warping the images with the velocity field as $\theta_0^w = \frac{1}{k}\sum_{i=1}^k I_i(\text{Exp}(-v(w_0)))$. This simplified formulation of the conditional maximum-likelihood is a result of Henderson's mixed-model [12] that simplifies when all observations are on a common grid. With this estimate of θ, we estimate the variance parameters by minimizing the double negative log-likelihood of the linearized model

$$\mathcal{L}(\sigma^2, S, C) = nk \log \sigma^2 + \sum_{i=1}^k \log \det V_i +$$
$$\frac{1}{\sigma^2} \sum_{i=1}^k (I_i - \theta^{wo} + Z_i w^0)^T V_i^{-1} (I_i - \theta^{wo} + Z_i w^0). \tag{2}$$

where $V_i = Z_i^T C_i Z_i + S + \mathbb{I}_i$. Computing (2) directly is computationally intractable. This is because the dimensionality of S, V is m^2, where m is the number of voxels in the image. We handle this by two assumptions: (a) The support of the kernel used to construct the covariance matrix of the spatial correlation effect is sufficiently large that the inverse of the covariance matrix resembles a block-diagonal matrix, see e.g. assumption [13]; and (b) the interaction between the blocks is negligible. This allows the likelihood to be approximated by an integral over smaller computationally tractable patches over the image. Therefore, (2) can be rewritten as:

$$\mathcal{L}(\sigma^2, S, C) \approx nk \log \sigma^2 + \sum_{i=1}^k \sum_{j=1}^p \log \det V_{i,j} +$$
$$\frac{1}{\sigma^2} \sum_{i=1}^k \sum_{j=1}^p (I_{i,j} - \theta^{wo} + Z_{i,j} w^0)^T V_{i,j}^{-1} (I_{i,j} - \theta_j^{wo} + Z_{i,j} w^0). \tag{3}$$

where $V_{i,j} = Z_{i,j}^T C_i Z_{i,j} + S_j + \mathbb{I}_j$. Here $j = 1 \ldots p$ is the patch number of the image with total p patches. The estimation process is now repeated: Given the current estimate of the template θ and the variance estimates, the new deformation parameters w^0 for the linearization point are chosen as the most likely predictions in the original non-linear model (1). That is, they are given by minimizing the negative log posterior of the deformation given the image data in model (1):

$$\mathcal{P}(w) = \sum_{i=1}^k \sum_{j=1}^p (I_{i,j} - \theta_j^{w_i})^T (S_j + I_j)^{-1} (I_{i,j} - \theta_j^{w_i}) + w_i^T C_i w_i. \tag{4}$$

To reconstruct the bias field for a given iteration, the conditional expectation of the spatially correlated effect x_i given the data I_i and the most likely deformation parameters w_i^0 are computed under the maximum likelihood estimates for the model parameters:

$$E[x_i | w_i^0, I_i] = S(S + I)^{-1}(I_i - \theta_j^{w_i}). \tag{5}$$

Note that the best linear unbiased predictor (BLUP) [14] of w_i in the linearized model given the image data I_i is realized by $E[w_i|I_i]$ which is computed as $(C_i^{-1} + Z_i^T(\mathbb{I}_i + S)^{-1}Z_i)^{-1}Z^T(\mathbb{I}_i + S)^{-1}(I_i - \theta^{w_i^0} + Zw_0^i)$.

3.1 Covariance Matrices

A key aspect of this statistical model is the choice of covariance matrices for the spatially correlated effects and the deformation effects. Current Bayesian methods model the inverse of the covariance matrix directly by the means of an operator; typically of the Cauchy-Navier type which takes the form, $L = -\alpha\nabla + \beta$ where ∇ is the Laplace operator. The parameter α here controls the smoothness of the covariance. In this paper, since we work with patches, it is more intuitive to model the covariance matrix directly. We model the covariance matrices for both the deformation parameters and the spatial correlation using Wendland kernels [15] that are compactly supported reproducing kernels. The covariance matrices are constructed using $C = \lambda^2 K(c_i, c_j)$, $\lambda \in (0, \infty)$, $K(a, b) = r^4(4r + 1)$, $r = (1 - t, 0)_+$, $t = \frac{||a-b||}{s}$, where c_i are the kernel centers.

For the spatially correlated effect $(S = \beta K)$, a similar representation is chosen. However, we choose the parametric subspace to be the same size as that of the image i.e., a kernel is centered at every voxel as opposed to the much smaller subspace spanned by the deformation kernels. The amplitude of these covariance matrices are controlled by parameters λ, β. These parameters are estimated by optimizing the likelihood (2). The smoothness of the deformation is controlled by C. We here keep C fixed though parameters of C, e.g. range and scale, can also be optimized for in (2).

3.2 Multi-scale Deformation Model

We model deformation fields as path of diffeomorphisms generated by integrating stationary velocity fields (SVFs). Let $G \subset \mathrm{Diff}(\Omega)$ be a Lie subgroup of the group of diffeomorphic transformations $\varphi : \Omega \to \Omega$, and let $\phi : \Omega \times \mathbb{R} \to \Omega$ be a path in G. Let V be the tangent space of G at identity Id containing velocity fields $v : \Omega \to \mathbb{R}^d$. In SVFs, the governing differential equation can be written as:

$$\frac{\partial\phi(\mathbf{x}, t)}{\partial t} = v(\phi(\mathbf{x}, t)), \quad \varphi = \phi(\mathbf{x}, 1) = \mathrm{Exp}(v). \qquad (6)$$

The final transformation ϕ is the Lie group exponential $\mathrm{Exp}(v)$. The integration in (6) can be numerically realized as an Euler integration. We use the kernel bundle framework [5,6] in this paper. In short, the concept of the space of velocity fields V is extended to a family $\hat{V}$ of spaces of velocity fields. The velocity fields are linear sums of individual kernels at R levels

$$v(\mathbf{x}) = \sum_{m=1}^{R} v_m = \sum_{m=1}^{R}\sum_{i}^{N_m} K_m(c_i^m, \mathbf{x})w_i^m. \qquad (7)$$

Here K is an interpolating Wendland kernel, R is the total number of kernel bundle levels, N_m is the number of kernels at each level and c is center of each kernel at the kernel bundle level. The parameter w^m is associated with the mth kernel bundle level, and we assume that $w_i^m \sim \mathcal{N}(0, \sigma^2 C^m)$, where C^m is the covariance matrix for each kernel bundle level with its distinct support and smoothness.

4   Experiments and Results

We perform an evaluation on the MGH10 dataset[1]. The dataset contains 10 images each with the dimension of $182 \times 218 \times 182$ and a voxel resolution of 1, 1.33, 1 mm. The images are initially co-registered rigidly. For bias recovery only a subset of 5 subjects is used.   One of the major challenges in the field of image

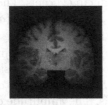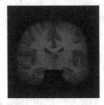

Fig. 1. An illustration of the image with bias field (left) and the recovered image (right).

template estimation is validation. Since the underlying geometry of the space of images is unknown, the definition of modes of populations is difficult. Therefore, the validation needs to be tied to specific applications of template estimation like image segmentation or even validation of the underlying image registrations. For the 2 experiments in this paper, we chose 3 kernel bundle levels each with a control point spacing of 20, 10, 6 mm respectively. The support of the kernel used to construct the covariance matrix for the deformations is fixed to 4 across the kernel bundle levels. The support of the spatial correlation variance kernel was set to 40. We perform 2 experiments to validate our template estimation method.

4.1   Bias Field Recovery

We select a subset of 5 images from the database and add artificial multiplicative bias to the image of form bias $= 1 + \exp(-\frac{x^2+y^2+z^2}{2*30^2}) * 0.05$. We then apply our statistical model to estimate the template and inspect whether the corrupted image can be recovered. As illustrated in Fig. 1 the image recovered is free of the bias field illustrating the robustness of the method towards scanner-related artifacts.

---

[1] www.mindboggle.info.

4.2   Template Estimation

In this paper, we evaluate the overlaps of segmentations of images mapped to the estimated template. This experiment was chosen to illustrate the performance of the underlying registration method in the paper. Figure 2 illustrates the mean and target overlaps estimated by mapping the 10 individual images to the template space and measuring pairwise overlaps. The overlaps are comparable to what state-of-the-art registration methods have obtained on the same dataset [16]. The kernel bundle scales are sequentially optimized. However, if one switches to a parallel optimization across scales, a significant improvement in the overlaps may be expected. Also in the illustration is the non-aligned template image and aligned template image. The sharpness of the template is particularly visible in corpus collosum.

To further demonstrate the effectiveness of the proposed template estimation method and benefits of multi-scale deformation, we visually inspect the atlas estimated in key regions like hippocampus and putamen. As illustrated in Fig. 2, as the kernel bundle resolution becomes finer, the sharper are the boundaries of the anatomical structure.

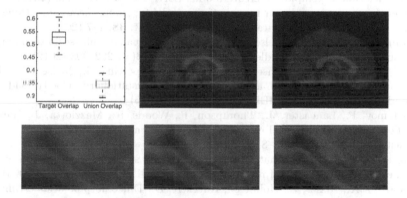

Fig. 2. Pairwise mean and target overlaps; Unaligned template and aligned template; Evolution of the appearance of hippocampus and putamen across kernel bundle scales (2 scales) with leftmost being the unaligned template.

5   Discussion and Conclusion

We presented a class of non-linear mixed effect models for estimating 3D brain templates, and we proposed to simultaneously estimate both bias field and deformation parameters in a data-driven maximum likelihood setting. In addition, we proposed to incorporate the kernel bundle framework in the random deformation effects to account for deformations occurring at different scales. We illustrated the application of our in both bias field correction and template estimation. The basis for the simultaneous estimation of the deformation and spatially correlated bias was results of [4] where the authors showed that estimation of deformation parameters is biased if the data is preprocessed first followed by the prediction of deformation parameters. We modeled deformations as random geodesics on the diffeomorphism group and estimated variance parameters of both the deformation and bias field from data instead of setting them ad-hoc. In future work, we will investigate replacing random geodesics by more geometrically natural distributions on the space of diffeomorphism [17]. An important next step for this work will be to extend the method to account for multiple population means.

References

1. Joshi, S., Davis, B., Jomier, M., Gerig, G.: Unbiased diffeomorphic atlas construction for computational anatomy. Neuroimage **23**, S151–S160 (2004)
2. Zhang, M., Singh, N., Fletcher, P.T.: Bayesian estimation of regularization and atlas building in diffeomorphic image registration. In: Gee, J.C., Joshi, S., Pohl, K.M., Wells, W.M., Zöllei, L. (eds.) IPMI 2013. LNCS, vol. 7917, pp. 37–48. Springer, Heidelberg (2013). doi:10.1007/978-3-642-38868-2_4
3. Allassonniere, S., Kuhn, E.: Stochastic algorithm for parameter estimation for dense deformable template mixture model. ESAIM-PS **14**, 382–408 (2010)
4. Raket, L., et al.: A nonlinear mixed-effects model for simultaneous smoothing and registration of functional data. Pattern Recogn. Lett. **38**, 1–7 (2014)
5. Sommer, S., Lauze, F., Nielsen, M., Pennec, X.: Sparse multi-scale dieomorphic registration: the kernel bundle framework. JMIV **46**(3), 292–308 (2012)
6. Pai, A., Sommer, S., Sorensen, L., Darkner, S., Sporring, J., Nielsen, M.: Kernel bundle diffeomorphic image registration using stationary velocity fields and Wendland basis functions. IEEE TMI **PP**(99) (2015)
7. Kochunov, P., Lancaster, J., Thompson, P., Woods, R., Mazziotta, J., Hardies, J., Fox, P.: Regional spatial normalization: toward an optimal target. J. Comput. Assist. Tomogr. **25**(5), 805–816 (2001)
8. Rueckert, D., et al.: Automatic construction of 3D statistical deformation models of the brain using non-rigid registration. IEEE TMI **22**(8), 1014–1025 (2003)
9. Vialard, F.X., Risser, L., Holm, D., Rueckert, D.: Diffeomorphic atlas estimation using Karcher mean and geodesic shooting on volumetric images. In: MIUA (2011)
10. Zöllei, L., Jenkinson, M., Timoner, S., Wells, W.: A marginalized MAP approach and EM optimization for pair-wise registration. In: Karssemeijer, N., Lelieveldt, B. (eds.) IPMI 2007. LNCS, vol. 4584, pp. 662–674. Springer, Heidelberg (2007). doi:10.1007/978-3-540-73273-0_55
11. Hromatka, M., Zhang, M., Fleishman, G.M., Gutman, B., Jahanshad, N., Thompson, P., Fletcher, P.T.: A hierarchical Bayesian model for multi-site diffeomorphic image atlases. In: Navab, N., Hornegger, J., Wells, W.M., Frangi, A.F. (eds.) MICCAI 2015. LNCS, vol. 9350, pp. 372–379. Springer, Cham (2015). doi:10.1007/978-3-319-24571-3_45
12. Henderson, C.R.: Estimation of genetic parameters. Biometrics **6**, 186–187 (1950)
13. Si, S., et al.: Memory efficient kernel approximation. In: ICML (2014)
14. Robinson, G.: That BLUP is a good thing: the estimation of random effects. Stat. Sci. **6**(1), 15–51 (1991)
15. Wendland, H.: Piecewise polynomial, positive definite and compactly supported radial functions of minimal degree. Adv. Comput. Math. **4**(1), 389–396 (1995)

16. Sommer, S.: Anisotropic distributions on manifolds: template estimation and most probable paths. In: Ourselin, S., Alexander, D.C., Westin, C.-F., Cardoso, M.J. (eds.) IPMI 2015. LNCS, vol. 9123, pp. 193–204. Springer, Cham (2015). doi:10.1007/978-3-319-19992-4_15
17. Sommer, S.: Anisotropic distributions on manifolds: template estimation and most probable paths. Information Processing in Medical Imaging 193–204(2015)

Bayesian Multiview Manifold Learning Applied to Hippocampus Shape and Clinical Score Data

Giorgos Sfikas[1([⊠])] and Christophoros Nikou[2]

[1] Computational Intelligence Laboratory,
Institute of Informatics and Telecommunications, NCSR "Demokritos",
Athens, Greece
sfikas@iit.demokritos.gr
[2] Department of Computer Science and Engineering,
University of Ioannina, Ioannina, Greece
cnikou@cs.uoi.gr

Abstract. In this paper, we present a novel Bayesian model for manifold learning, suitable for data that are comprised of multiple modes of observations. Our data are assumed to be lying on a non-linear, low-dimensional manifold, modelled as a locally linear structure. The manifold local structure and the manifold coordinates are latent stochastic variables that are estimated from a training set. Through the use of appropriate prior distributions, neighbouring points are constrained to have similar manifold coordinates as well as similar manifold geometry. A single set of latent coordinates is learned, common for all views. We show how to solve the model with variational inference. We also exploit the multiview aspect of the proposed model, by showing how to estimate missing views of unseen data. We have tested the proposed model and methods on medical imaging data of the OASIS brain MRI dataset [6]. The data are comprised of four views: two views that correspond to clinical scores and two views that correspond to hippocampus shape extracted from the OASIS MR images. Our model is successfully used to map the multimodal data to probabilistic embedding coordinates, as well as estimate missing clinical scores and shape information of test data.

1 Introduction

Using low-dimensional structures to model data is a widely used and studied practice in the context of a vast range of problems. Methods that deal with low-dimensional modeling may assume either a linear or a non-linear structure of data. Linear models like principal component analysis (PCA), are naturally simpler and more straightforward in their application. Non-linear models on the other hand, allow a more accurate and flexible representation of the data structure. A wealth of models exists for non-linear dimensionality reduction, or otherwise known as (non-linear) manifold learning [4].

Manifold modeling techniques typically treat data and model parameters as deterministic (in the sense of being non-probabilistic). The linear PCA algorithm, as well as the closely related canonical correlation analysis (CCA), have

© Springer International Publishing AG 2017
H. Müller et al. (Eds.): MCV/BAMBI 2016, LNCS 10081, pp. 160–171, 2017.
DOI: 10.1007/978-3-319-61188-4_15

been shown to be expressible as equivalent probabilistic models [1,2]. In terms of probabilistic PCA/CCA, the latent variable acts as an embedding coordinate vector. In [1], a graphical model was introduced that was proved to be equivalent to CCA. Both models can be solved with Expectation-Maximization (EM) [2]. Interestingly, in both probabilistic models a single set of normally distributed latent variables is defined, while they differ in that probabilistic CCA defines two, instead of a single one, sets of observed variables (*views* in CCA parlance) and two sets of projections from the common latent space to the view spaces.

Non-linear manifold learning schemes are typically deterministic in the way they treat data and parameters, with few extensions to probabilistic models. One exception to this rule is the recently proposed locally linear latent variable model (LL-LVM) [7]. LL-LVM employs a probabilistic graphical model to describe observations, manifold coordinates and tangents [7]. The manifold is defined in terms of a patchwork of locally linear subspaces, that are represented using the tangent space to each point. The model is solved with standard variational inference (VI) [2]. LL-LVM is closely related to the Gaussian Process Latent Variable Model (GP-LVM) [5].

Manifold modeling has been extensively used in medical imaging in the recent years [4,10]. In [4], manifolds are learned on sets of brain structural MR images. New brain images are projected onto the manifold and a regression model is proposed, linking the MRI structure with subject clinical scores. In [10], an embedding is learned over brain MRIs that is used for atlas propagation. Registering one image to another is broken down to a set of subsequent registrations, following the shortest path over the learned manifold.

In this paper, we present a novel Bayesian model for manifold learning that can handle multiple observed views. Views here are to be understood as different sets of observations or different modes of measurements per observed datum, with each view typically having different dimensionality and statistics. This setup is in contrast to standard manifold learning techniques that typically assume a single source of observations and a non-probabilistic setup. In the same way that probabilistic CCA can be viewed as probabilistic PCA with multiple outputs [1], hence generalizing linear manifold learning to multiple views, the current model extends the LL-LVM model of [7]. Under this consideration we name the proposed model multiview locally linear latent variable model (MLL-LVM), underpinning its relation with LL-LVM. The proposed model is solved using variational inference. We show that a set of useful operations like out-of-sample extensions, predicting missing views, and generating new observations given the embedding coordinates, are all naturally defined in terms of the Bayesian model.

In a nutshell, from a theoretical point of view the novel characteristics of the proposed model compared to LL-LVM [7] are: (a) An extension of the model to handle more than a single view/mode of observation, (b) derivation of VI updates for the extended model and (c) derivation of the required formulae to estimate missing views given observed views. Note that the latter point is only compatible with the present model and not with LL-LVM or other single-view models, since it applies only to a scenario where we have more than one view.

The proposed model is successfully applied in a medical imaging context, where various shape data and clinical ratings from a set of Alzheimer's Disease (AD) and controls are used to learn common latent manifold coordinates. Brain MR images are used to extract shape information about subject left and right hippocampi, which alongside clinical scores make up the set of observed views. All views, despite being heterogenous and following different statistics, are hence treated in a unified manner with our model. Also importantly, all estimates (out-of-sample coordinates, missing views) are computed in the form of posterior probability density functions, since the model is fully Bayesian.

The remainder of this paper is structured as follows. In Sect. 2, we present the proposed multi-view Bayesian model, we show how to solve it using variational inference, and show how to estimate missing views. In Sect. 3, we train our model on the OASIS data set and estimate unknown clinical scores and hippocampus shapes given the observed subject views. In Sect. 4, we discuss final conclusions and thoughts about the perspective of the proposed work.

2   Methods

The basis of the proposed method is a novel Bayesian model, trained on a set multimodal data of N observations and V views. After training, the model can be used on new data in order to estimate one or more of their views that may be missing. In this section, we present the proposed observational model, we show how to solve it with VI, and derive the formulae required to predict missing views.

2.1   Generative Model

Observed data: The input to our model is a set of observations y and a graph $\mathcal{G}$. Each observation y^n of the observation set y is itself a set of V observed views $y^n = \{y_1^n, y_2^n, \cdots, y_V^n\}$, with each view being a set of elements with corresponding per-view dimensionality $d_{y_1}, d_{y_2}, \cdots, d_{y_V}$. N observed elements correspond to each of the V views, and for view v we have $\{y_v^1, y_v^2, \cdots, y_v^N\}$.

The graph $\mathcal{G}$ contains one node for each observation, and an edge exists between nodes (n,m) if and only if y^n and y^m are neighbours. A symmetric $N \times N$ adjacency matrix G corresponds to the graph structure of $\mathcal{G}$, with $G=[\eta^{nm}]$. Element $[\eta^{nm}]_{n=1..N, m=1..N}$ is equal to one if observations n and m are neighbours, otherwise it is zero.

In the assumed application context, each patient appears as a single observation y^n for the model, and each view corresponds to a different type of measurement for the patient. For example, for the nth patient, y_1^n may contain brain MRI T1 data, y_2^n a scalar clinical rating and y_3^n a brain connectogram. Patients that are similar enough with respect to the available measurements are recorded as neighbours in $\mathcal{G}$.

The graphical representation for the proposed generative model can be examined in Fig. 1. Note that a single set of embedding coordinates x are defined,

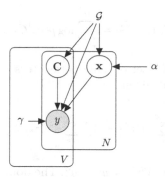

Fig. 1. The graphical model for the proposed MLL-LVM. V views are assumed for N observed data points. The latent variables x are embedding coordinates, common for all views. Latent variables C model the relation of the embedding coordinates x with each separate observed view. $\mathcal{G}$ is the fixed neighbourhood structure. γ and α are deterministic parameters that control the form of the likelihood function and the form of the prior on latent embedding coordinates respectively.

common for all views, while manifold geometry C and observations y are view-specific. In terms of the graphical model, this is the basic difference between the proposed model and LL-LVM [7]. The latter can be seen as a special case of our model, for $V = 1$.

Assumed distributions and relations with latent variables: Embedding coordinates can be concatenated to a single vector $x = \lfloor x^{1 \, T} \, x^{2 \, T} \cdots x^{N \, T} \rfloor^{T}$, where $x \in \mathcal{R}^{d_x N}$. The prior on latent variables x constraints elements that are neighbours to have embedding coordinates that lie close to each other:

$$\log p(x|G, \alpha) = -\frac{1}{2} \sum_{n=1}^{N} (\alpha \|x^n\|^2 + \sum_{m=1}^{N} \eta^{nm} \|x^n - x^m\|^2) + const. \quad (1)$$

The set of linear projections that correspond to the vth view can be concatenated to a single matrix $C_v = [C_v^1 C_v^2 \cdots C_v^N]$, where $C_v \in \mathcal{R}^{d_{y_v} \times d_x N}$. For all sets of linear maps C_v, a prior is defined that constrains neighbouring maps to be close to each other in the sense of the Frobenius norm:

$$\log p(C_v|G) = -\frac{\epsilon}{2} \|\sum_{n=1}^{N} C_v^n\|_F^2 - \frac{1}{2} \sum_{n=1}^{N} \sum_{m=1}^{N} \eta^{nm} \|C_v^n - C_v^m\|_F^2 + const. \quad (2)$$

where ϵ is set to a constant, small value. Local manifold tangents of neighbouring points are equivalently constrained to be similar, favouring smooth solutions with low-curvature for all views.

Observed views are assumed to be conditionally independent given x. Hence the model likelihood is defined as the sum of V terms, each corresponding to a different view:

$$\log p(y|C, x, \gamma, G) = \sum_{v=1}^{V} \log p(y_v|C_v, x, \gamma_v, G) \tag{3}$$

where $\gamma = \gamma_1, \gamma_2, \cdots, \gamma_V$ is a set of scale parameters. The log-likelihood component specific to each view is given by:

$$\log p(y_v|C_v, x, \gamma_v, G) = -\frac{\epsilon}{2}\|\sum_{n=1}^{N} y_v^n\|^2 - \frac{1}{2}\sum_{n=1}^{N}\sum_{m=1}^{N} \eta^{nm}\gamma_v\|\Delta_{y_v}^{m,n} - C_v^n \Delta_x^{m,n}\|^2 + const. \tag{4}$$

where $\Delta_x^{m,n} = x^m - x^n$ and $\Delta_{y_v}^{m,n} = y_v^m - y_v^n$. The double-summation term in the above equation encodes the assertion that $C_v^n \Delta_{x_v}^{m,n} \approx \Delta_{y_v}^{m,n}$, or that the assumed manifolds are locally linear.

Following [7], it is straightforward to show that x and $y_v \ \forall v \in [1..V]$ are normally distributed, and $C_v \ \forall v \in [1..V]$ follow the matrix-normal distribution. More specifically,

$$x|G, \alpha \sim \mathcal{N}(0, \Sigma_x^0), \tag{5}$$

$$C_v|G \sim \mathcal{MN}(0, I_{d_{y_v}}, \Sigma_{C_v}^0), \forall v \in [1..V], \tag{6}$$

$$y_v|C_v, x, \gamma_v, G \sim \mathcal{N}(\mu_{y_v}^0, \Sigma_{y_v}^0), \forall v \in [1..V], \tag{7}$$

where for $\Sigma_x^{-1} = \alpha I_{d_x N} + 2L \otimes I_{d_x}$ and $L = diag(G1_N) - G$ is the graph Laplacian matrix of G. The prior covariance $\Sigma_C^{0}{}^{-1} = \epsilon JJ^T + 2L \otimes I_{d_x}$ is the same for all view distributions. The likelihood parameters are $\Sigma_{y_v}^{0}{}^{-1} = (\epsilon 1_N 1_N^T + 2\gamma_v L) \otimes I_{d_{y_v}}$, $\mu_{y_v}^0 = \Sigma_{y_v}^0 e_v$, where $e_v = [e_v^{1T}, e_v^{1T}, \cdots, e_v^{NT}]^T \in \mathcal{R}^{d_{y_v} N}$, $e_v^n = -\sum_{m=1}^{N} \eta^{mn}\gamma_v(C_v^m + C_v^n)\Delta_x^{m,n}$.

2.2 Solution with Variational Inference

Solving the model amounts to calculating the posterior distributions for the shared coordinates x and the sets of linear projections $C_v, \forall v \in [1..V]$, as well as the non-stochastic parameters $\{\gamma_v\}_{v=1}^V$ and α. As an exact calculation of the posterior is intractable, we employ variational inference [2] to approximate it. In VI, the model is solved by iterating between optimizing the Kullback-Leibler divergence $KL(q\|p)$ of the posterior estimate q and the actual posterior p, and optimizing a lower bound $\mathcal{L}$ of the model likelihood. In our model, the variational lower bound $\mathcal{L}$ is defined as

$$\mathcal{L}(q, C, x, \gamma, \alpha) = \int_{C,x} q(C, x) \log \frac{p(y, C, x|G, \gamma, \alpha)}{q(C, x)} dCdx. \tag{8}$$

According to VI theory, the posteriors of the latent variables are estimated by taking expectations of the model joint distribution, in our case $p(C, x|\mathcal{G}, \gamma, \alpha)$, over all latent variables except the one that is being computed. Formally, for the approximate posteriors $q^*(x), q^*(C_1), q^*(C_2), \cdots, q^*(C_V)$ we have

$$\log q^*(x) = <\log p(y, C, x|G, \gamma, \alpha)>_C + const. \tag{9}$$

$$\log q^*(C_v) = <\log p(y, C, x|G, \gamma, \alpha)>_{x, C_1, \cdots, C_{v-1}, C_{v+1}, \cdots, C_V} + const., \forall v \in [1..V] \quad (10)$$

Key to model tractability with VI is the fact that the log-likelihood term (Eq. 4) can be written as a quadratic function in both x and C. More specifically,

$$\log p(y|C, x, \gamma, G) = -\frac{1}{2}[x^T \{\sum_{v=1}^{V} A_v\} x - 2x^T \{\sum_{v=1}^{V} b_v\}] + Z_x, \quad (11)$$

$$= -\frac{1}{2} \sum_{v=1}^{V} Tr[\Gamma_v C_v^T C_v - 2\gamma_v C_v^T H] + Z_C \quad (12)$$

where we followed [7] in a related calculation, and Z_x, Z_C contain terms not depending on x or C respectively. Matrix A_v is of size $Nd_x \times Nd_x$ and b_v is of size $Nd_x \times 1$. Matrix Γ_v is of size $Nd_x \times Nd_x$. Hence all priors x, $C_1, C_2, \cdots, C_V$ are conjugate to the likelihood and VI is tractable.

Variational E step update of $q(x)$: Equation (9) can be further decomposed to

$$\log q^*(x) = <\log p(y|C, x, \gamma, G)>_C + \log p(x|G, \alpha) + const.$$

$$= -\frac{1}{2} \sum_{v=1}^{V} [x^T A_v x - 2x^T b_v] - \frac{1}{2}[x^T \Sigma_x^{-1(0)}] + const.$$

where we have used Eqs. (5) and (11). As the non-constant terms are quadratic in x, the approximate posterior of x is Gaussian. Thus we have $q^*(x) = \mathcal{N}(x|\mu_x, \Sigma_x)$ with

$$\Sigma_x^{-1} = \Sigma_x^{-1(0)} + \sum_{v=1}^{V} <A_v>_{C_v}, \quad (13)$$

$$\mu_x - <x> = \Sigma_x \sum_{v=1}^{V} <b_v>_{C_v}. \quad (14)$$

We also calculate the expectation $<xx^T>$, useful for some later updates,

$$<x^n x^{mT}> = \Sigma_x^{nm} + <x^n><x^m>^T, \quad (15)$$

where Σ_x^{nm} is the $(n, m)^{th}$ chunk of size $d_x \times d_x$ of this matrix. Expectations for A_v and b_v can be derived following a related calculation in [7]. We show updates for all $d_x \times d_x$-sized chunks of the $Nd_x \times Nd_x$-sized matrix A_v, and updates for all d_x-sized chunks of the Nd_x-sized matrix b_v:

$$<A_v^{nm}>_{C_v} = \gamma_v^2 \sum_{p=1}^{N} \sum_{q=1}^{N} \{[\hat{L}_v^{pq} - \hat{L}_v^{pm} - \hat{L}_v^{nq} + \hat{L}_v^{nm}]\eta^{pn}\eta^{qm}$$

$$\times <C_v^{pT} C_v^q + C_v^{pT} C_v^m + C_v^{nT} C_v^q + C_v^{nT} C_v^m>_{C_v}\}, \quad (16)$$

$$<b_v^n>_{C_v} = \gamma_v \sum_{m=1}^{N} \eta^{nm} \{<C_v^m>^T (y_v^n - y_v^m) - <C_v^n>^T (y_v^m - y_v^n)\}, \quad (17)$$

where the quantity $\hat{L}_v$ for each v is equal to $(\epsilon 11^T + 2\gamma_v L)^{-1}$.

Variational E step update of $q(C_v)$, $v \in [1..V]$: We decompose Eq. (10) as:

$$\log q^*(C_v) = -\frac{1}{2}\sum_{v=1}^{V} Tr[\Gamma_v C_v^T C_v - 2\gamma_v C_v^T H] + \mathcal{MN}(0, I_{d_{y_v}}, \Sigma_C^0) + const., \quad (18)$$

where we wrote the likelihood function in terms of C_v using Eq. (12). The approximate posterior distribution for the vth view projection matrix C_v can thus be written as a matrix normal distribution $q^*(C_v) = \mathcal{MN}(\mu_{C_v}, I_{d_{y_v}}, \Sigma_{C_v})$ with

$$\Sigma_{C_v}^{-1} = \Sigma_{C_v}^{-1(0)} + <\Gamma_v>_x, \quad (19)$$

$$<C_v^{nT}C_v^m>_x = <C_v^n>_x^T <C_v^m>_x + d_y \Sigma_{C_v}^{nm}, \quad (20)$$

where $\Sigma_{C_v}^{nm}$ is the $(n, m)^{th}$ chunk of size $d_x \times d_x$, and C_v^n is the nth chunk of the respective matrices. Also,

$$\mu_{C_v} = <C_v>_x = \gamma <H_v>_x \Sigma_{C_v}. \quad (21)$$

Finally, expectations for quantities Γ_v and H_v are given as:

$$<\Gamma_v^{nm}>_x = \gamma_v^2 \sum_{p=1}^{N}\sum_{q=1}^{N}\{[\hat{L}_v^{pq} - \hat{L}_v^{pm} - \hat{L}_v^{nq} + \hat{L}_v^{nm}]\eta^{pn}\eta^{qm}$$

$$\times <x^p x^{qT} - x^p x^{mT} - x^n x^{qT} + x^n x^{mT}>_x\}, \quad (22)$$

$$<H_v^n>_x = \sum_{m=1}^{N}\eta^{nm}(y_v^m <x^m>_x^T - y_v^m <x^n>_x^T - y_v^m <x^m>_x^T + y_v^m <x^n>_x^T). \quad (23)$$

Variational M step update of α, γ_v, $\forall v \in [1..V]$: In the maximization step we optimize the variation lower bound with respect to non-stochastic parameters α and γ_v, $\forall v \in [1..V]$. The update of α is identical to the one for the single-view case [7]. The update for γ_v is similar to the update for γ of [7], save that for each view it is now calculated over y_v and the statistics of C_v instead of y and C respectively.

We alternate the aforementioned E-step updates for the approximate posterior of x (Eqs. 13–17), the approximate posterior of C (Eqs. 19–23) and M-step updates until convergence.

2.3   Estimation of Missing Views for New Data

Given a previously unseen datum y^{new} for which only part of all the V views are observed, we can use the trained model to estimate the missing views. In order to do this, first we add the new datum to the training set and re-compute the E-step for the new datum only, keeping posteriors for the original trained data and deterministic parameters fixed. The new observation is added to the previous graph structure by computing its nearest neighbours. Using the E-step equations gives us an estimate of the posterior distributions $q(x^{new})$ and $q(C^{new})$ for the new datum. These steps let us effectively project the new observation onto the manifold, a process known in the literature as out-of-sample projection [7].

The set of missing views $\hat{v}$ of y^{new} are treated also as latent variables, for which we require their approximate posterior distribution $q(y)$. Hence the joint posterior now also includes $q(\{y_v^{new}\}_{v\in\hat{v}})$, decomposed using the mean field approximation [2] into $\{q(y_v^{new})\}_{v\in\hat{v}}$. In order to estimate the posterior for missing view v, we compute the expectation of the model evidence. This is formally written as

$$logq^*(y_v^{new}) = <logp(y_v, C_v, x|G, \gamma_v, \alpha)>_{x,C_v} +const. \tag{24}$$

The above equation, combined with the likelihood formula (Eq. 4), where we have kept all observations fixed except y^{new}, gives a posterior Normal distribution $\mathcal{N}(y_v^{new}|m_v^{new}, S_v^{new})$ with statistics given by

$$S_v^{new} = (2\gamma_v \sum_{m-1}^{N} \eta^{m,new} + \epsilon)^{-1} I_{d_{y_v}} \tag{25}$$

$$m_v^{new} = S_v^{new}(2\gamma_v \sum_{m=1}^{N} \{\eta^{m,new}[y^n + 1/2(<C_v^{new}> + <C_v^m>)<\Delta_x^{new,m}>]\} - \frac{\epsilon}{2}\sum_{m-1}^{N} y_v^m) \tag{26}$$

In summary, in order to estimate the missing views of an unseen datum y^{new} we iterate through the E- step updates for the approximate posterior of x^{new} (Eqs. 13–17), the approximate posterior of C^{new} (Eqs. 19–23) and the approximate posterior for y^{new} (Eqs. 25 and 26), keeping fixed the deterministic model parameters and all other point posteriors[1].

3   Experiments

3.1   Dataset

We have experimented with data from the OASIS database [6]. In our evaluation we have included the 198 subjects aged 60 or more found in the cross-sectional set of OASIS. 100 of these subjects have been diagnosed with very mild to moderate AD. The rest of the subjects are used as controls. We have used in total 4 views/modes for each subject. The two first views are the clinical scores Minimental State Exam (MMSE) and Clinical Dementia Rating (CDR). The other two views correspond to shape information for the left and the right hippocampus of each subject respectively. The volumetric characteristics of the hippocampus are known to be correlated with the advance of AD [9].

In order to create the shape views, we have first segmented the OASIS T1-modulated MR images with Freesurfer [3]. We have then computed deformation

---

[1] MATLAB code that implements training and missing view estimation using the presented model is available at https://github.com/sfikas/mll-lvm/.

fields for each volume, given as the output of matching with an in-set template image. The template, one for each hippocampus, was chosen as the medoid image within the sets of left and right hippocampi. The medoid was taken with respect to a distance metric that is analogous to the total magnitude of the deformation field required to perform a matching non-rigid deformation between volumes [4]. Deformation fields are subsampled to 25% of the original length of each axis, resulting in $11 \times 15 \times 8$ and $12 \times 14 \times 9$-sized fields of $\mathcal{R}^3$ vectors. These volumes are further vectorized into descriptors of 3960 and 4536 dimensions respectively.

We partitioned our dataset into a training set and a test set. The training set was used to learn the parameters of our model, and the test set was used to evaluate the model. We assigned the first 80% of the data (first in the sense of lexicographical OASIS id order) to the training set, and the rest to the test set. Mean clinical scores for both training and test differ by less than 10^{-2} (CDR) and 0.5 (MMSE) to the respective statistics of the full set (CDR $= 0.2$ and MMSE $= 27$ respectively).

3.2   Experimental Setup

Before proceeding to any tests we computed the neighbourhood structure G. To this end, a distance ζ^{nm} for all pairs of subjects (n, m) in the training set was first calculated. This distance fusions view-specific distances are $\zeta^{nm} = \sum_{v=1}^{V} \zeta_v^{nm}$. The view-specific distances are Euclidean distances over normalized view data. We computed embeddings with $d_x = 2$, which can be examined in Fig. 2, along with an overlay of clinical score values.

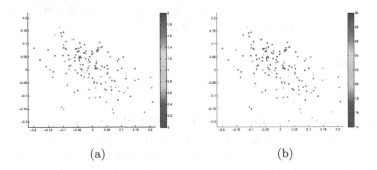

(a)   (b)

Fig. 2. Computed embedding given clinical score and shape information of the training data ($N = 158$ subjects). Approximate posterior mean values for x are shown, per subject. Point colours correspond to (a) CDR scores (b) MMSE scores. (Color figure online)

Estimating clinical scores given shape data: In the first experiment, we assumed that only shape information (views 3 and 4) was known for the test set subjects. For each test subject, we estimate the posterior distribution of its clinical scores (views

Table 1. Clinical score estimation given hippocampus shape data. We show the moments of the Gaussian posterior distribution of the clinical scores (mean ± st.deviation) for all the 40 test set subjects. Significant statistical correlation is reported between estimate means and ground truth for both CDR and MMSE (bottom row).

OASIS id	CDR		MMSE	
	Estimate	Actual	Estimate	Actual
Control subjects				
363	0.16 ± 0.32	0.00	28.3 ± 4.0	30.0
365	0.41 ± 0.32	0.00	24.4 ± 4.0	30.0
369	0.23 ± 0.05	0.00	27.3 ± 0.7	28.0
371	0.22 ± 0.07	0.00	27.6 ± 0.9	30.0
373	0.16 ± 0.32	0.00	28.4 ± 4.0	30.0
374	0.16 ± 0.32	0.00	28.3 ± 4.0	29.0
380	0.16 ± 0.32	0.00	28.3 ± 4.0	29.0
382	0.16 ± 0.32	0.00	27.8 ± 4.0	28.0
388	0.27 ± 0.09	0.00	26.8 ± 1.1	29.0
390	0.16 ± 0.32	0.00	27.3 ± 4.0	28.0
398	0.21 ± 0.10	0.00	27.9 ± 1.2	29.0
399	0.41 ± 0.32	0.00	26.9 ± 4.0	29.0
400	0.23 ± 0.07	0.00	27.0 ± 0.8	30.0
402	0.22 ± 0.11	0.00	27.4 ± 1.3	29.0
404	0.18 ± 0.10	0.00	28.0 ± 1.2	28.0
405	0.16 ± 0.32	0.00	28.4 ± 4.0	30.0
411	0.41 ± 0.32	0.00	27.4 ± 4.0	26.0
AD subjects				
418	0.66 ± 0.32	1.00	20.8 ± 4.0	20.0
422	0.16 ± 0.09	0.50	27.8 ± 1.1	29.0
423	0.16 ± 0.32	0.50	26.3 ± 4.0	18.0
424	0.28 ± 0.23	1.00	25.9 ± 2.8	15.0
425	0.41 ± 0.13	1.00	26.1 ± 1.6	22.0
426	0.24 ± 0.19	0.50	28.0 ± 2.3	24.0
428	0.66 ± 0.32	1.00	24.4 ± 4.0	29.0
430	0.41 ± 0.32	0.50	23.4 ± 4.0	25.0
432	0.67 ± 0.32	0.50	26.3 ± 4.0	30.0
438	0.16 ± 0.32	1.00	27.9 ± 4.0	23.0
440	0.32 ± 0.10	0.50	27.4 ± 1.2	29.0
441	0.18 ± 0.10	0.50	27.7 ± 1.2	28.0
445	0.29 ± 0.23	1.00	28.3 ± 2.8	20.0
446	0.41 ± 0.32	1.00	24.8 ± 4.0	23.0
447	0.41 ± 0.32	1.00	22.3 ± 4.0	17.0
449	0.23 ± 0.12	0.50	27.0 ± 1.5	26.0
451	0.32 ± 0.19	0.50	26.0 ± 2.3	27.0
452	0.41 ± 0.32	0.50	28.4 ± 4.0	29.0
453	0.41 ± 0.32	0.50	26.4 ± 4.0	24.0
454	0.16 ± 0.32	0.50	28.4 ± 4.0	27.0
455	0.25 ± 0.19	1.00	27.9 ± 2.3	22.0
456	0.16 ± 0.23	0.50	28.1 ± 2.8	29.0
457	0.16 ± 0.32	0.50	27.9 ± 4.0	23.0
	r	p-value	r	p-value
corr.coeff.	**0.43**	**0.006**	**0.44**	**0.004**

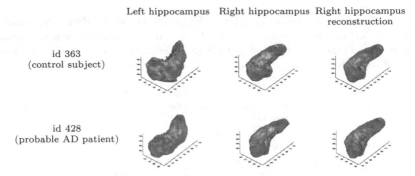

Fig. 3. Estimation of the right hippocampus given the left hippocampus shape data. We show reconstructions for a probable AD patient as well as for a control subject. Left column: Left hippocampus shapes on which the estimate is conditioned. Middle column: Right hippocampus ground truth data, shown here for comparison. Right column: Right hippocampus posterior mean, calculated with the proposed algorithm.

1 and 2), using the method described in Sect. 2.3. In order to fit the new datum onto the neighbourhood structure $\mathcal{G}$, we assigned neighbours according to a distance threshold chosen so that the mean number of neighbours is closest to $k = 5$. Data without neighbours are assigned their nearest neighbour to their neighbourhood.

We can see an overview of the results in Table 1. Note that all estimates are computed as posterior probability density functions. The moments of the posterior Gaussians are reported for all test set subjects, alongside with the ground truth values. The correlation coefficient between estimate mean values and ground truth is also computed. The results clearly indicate that there is statistically significant correlation between estimates and actual values. This result agrees with the fact, known from the related literature, that hippocampus shape and the progression of neurogenerative diseases such as AD are correlated [4], hence validating the usefulness of the proposed MLL-LVM model. Furthermore, our results come all in the form of pdfs, measuring estimation uncertainty in a natural and principled manner, in line with the model assumptions.

Estimating shape data given shape data: We have experimented with using the proposed model to calculate an estimate of missing shape data given existing shape data. To this end, we have trained our model with the set of left and right hippocampus shape data. We have assumed that the test set now contains information only about the left hippocampus. In other words, for the 40 images of the test we now assume only the right hippocampus shape view as available, while the left hippocampus shape is missing. We have calculated posterior distribution approximations of the right hippocampus shape given the model and the observed test left hippocampus. We show visual results in Fig. 3. The results show that the estimate right hippocampus is reasonably similar to the ground truth right hippocampus. Again, estimates are computed in the form of pdfs. Here however we show only mean volumes, due to visualization constraints.

4 Conclusion

We have presented a novel Bayesian model for manifold learning, and tested it on a set of medical data. The model assumes that observed values are comprised of a number of heterogenous views. The solution has been shown to be feasible with approximate inference. The proposed model also allows new test data to have one or more of their views missing; we have shown how to compute estimates of these views, in a manner that is consistent with the definition of model. All estimates are computed in the form of posterior probability distributions.

In perspective, the model can be used with any number and combination of modes. Other imaging modalities could be used as modes, or other descriptors that characterize other parts of the brain. Extensions of the probabilistic model could also be considered. For example, replacing the binary neighbourhood graph with a more flexible alternative could be envisaged, in the spirit of the continuous line process model of [8].

References

1. Bach, F.R., Jordan, M.I.: A probabilistic interpretation of canonical correlation analysis. Technical Report 688, Department of Statistics, University of California, Berkeley (2005)
2. Bishop, C.M.: Pattern Recogn. Mach. Learn. Springer, New York (2006)
3. Fischl, B.: FreeSurfer. Neuroimage 62(2), 774–781 (2012)
4. Gerber, S., Tasdizen, T., Fletcher, P.T., Joshi, S., Whitaker, R.: Alzheimers disease neuroimaging initiative. manifold modeling for brain population analysis. Med. Image Anal. 14(5), 643–653 (2010)
5. Lawrence, N.D.: Gaussian process latent variable models for visualisation of high dimensional data. Adv. Neural Inf. Process. Syst. 16(3), 329–336 (2004)
6. Marcus, D.S., Wang, T.H., Parker, J., Csernansky, J.G., Morris, J.C., Buckner, R.L.: Open access series of imaging studies (OASIS): cross-sectional MRI data in young, middle aged, nondemented, and demented older adults. J. Cogn. Neurosci. 19(9), 1498–1507 (2007)
7. Park, M., Jitkrittum, W., Qamar, A., Szabó, Z., Buesing, L., Sahani, M.: Bayesian manifold learning: the locally linear latent variable model (LL-LVM). In: Advances in Neural Information Processing Systems, pp. 154–162 (2015)
8. Sfikas, G., Nikou, C., Galatsanos, N., Heinrich, C.: Spatially varying mixtures incorporating line processes for image segmentation. J. Math. Imaging Vis. 36(2), 91–110 (2010)
9. Wang, L., Swank, J.S., Glick, I.E., Gado, M.H., Miller, M.I., Morris, J.C., Csernansky, J.G.: Changes in hippocampal volume and shape across time distinguish dementia of the Alzheimer type from healthy aging. Neuroimage 20(2), 667–682 (2003)
10. Wolz, R., Aljabar, P., Hajnal, J.V., Hammers, A., Rueckert, D.: Alzheimer's disease neuroimaging initiative: LEAP: learning embeddings for atlas propagation. NeuroImage 49(2), 1316–1325 (2010)

Rigid Slice-To-Volume Medical Image Registration Through Markov Random Fields

Roque Porchetto[1], Franco Stramana[1], Nikos Paragios[2], and Enzo Ferrante[2(✉)]

[1] UNICEN University, Tandil, Argentina
[2] CVN, CentraleSupelec-INRIA, Universite Paris-Saclay,
Châtenay-Malabry, France
ferrante.enzo@gmail.com

Abstract. Rigid slice-to-volume registration is a challenging task, which finds application in medical imaging problems like image fusion for image guided surgeries and motion correction for volume reconstruction. It is usually formulated as an optimization problem and solved using standard continuous methods. In this paper, we discuss how this task be formulated as a discrete labeling problem on a graph. Inspired by previous works on discrete estimation of linear transformations using Markov Random Fields (MRFs), we model it using a pairwise MRF, where the nodes are associated to the rigid parameters, and the edges encode the relation between the variables. We compare the performance of the proposed method to a continuous formulation optimized using simplex, and we discuss how it can be used to further improve the accuracy of our approach. Promising results are obtained using a monomodal dataset composed of magnetic resonance images (MRI) of a beating heart.

1 Introduction

Slice-to-volume registration has received increasing attention during the last decades within the medical imaging community. Given a tomographic 2D slice and a 3D volume as input, this challenging problem consists in finding the slice (extracted from the input volume and specified by an arbitrary rigid transformation) that best matches the 2D input image. We stress the fact that we are working with 2D slices (e.g. ultrasound (US)) as opposed to projective 2D images (e.g. X-ray images). This is important since both problems are usually refereed as 2D/3D registration, even if they are intrinsically different. In slice-to-volume registration, every pixel from the 2D image corresponds to a single voxel in 3D space. However, in a projective 2D image every pixel represents a projection of voxels from a given viewpoint.

One can formulate different versions of slice-to-volume registration, depending on several aspects of the problem such as the *matching criterion* used to determine the similarity between the images, the *transformation model* we aim at estimating, the *optimization strategy* used to infer the optimal transformation model (continuous or discrete) and the *number of slices* given as input. In this work, we propose an iconic method (where the matching criterion is defined as

© Springer International Publishing AG 2017
H. Müller et al. (Eds.): MCV/BAMBI 2016, LNCS 10081, pp. 172–185, 2017.
DOI: 10.1007/978-3-319-61188-4_16

a function of the image intensity values) to infer rigid transformation models (specified using 6-DOF). The input consists of a single slice and a single volume, and we formulate it as a discrete optimization problem.

Discrete methods, where the tasks are usually formulated as a discrete labeling problem on a graph, have become a popular strategy to model vision problems [24] (and particularly, biomedical vision problems [19]) thanks to their modularity, efficiency, robustness and theoretical simplicity. This paper presents a graph-based formulation (inspired by the work of [26,27]) to solve rigid (only) slice-to-volume registration using discrete methods. As we will discuss in Sect. 1.2, other works have tackled similar problems. However, to date, no work has shown the potential of discrete methods to deal with rigid slice-to-volume registration. Our main contribution is to put a new spin on graph-based registration theory, by demonstrating that discrete methods and graphical models are suitable to estimate rigid transformations mapping slice-to-volume. We validate our approach using a dataset of magnetic resonance images (MRI) of the heart, and we compare its performance with a state-of-the-art approach based on continuous optimization using simplex method. Moreover, in the spirit of encouraging reproducible research, we make the source code of the application publicly available at the following website: https://gitlab.com/franco.stramana1/slice-to-volume.

1.1 Motivation

In the extensive literature of medical image registration, it is possible to identify two main problems which motivated the development of slice-to-volume registration methods during the last decades. The first one is the fusion of pre-operative high-definition volumetric images with intra-operative tomographic slices to perform diagnostic and minimally invasive surgeries. In this case, slice-to-volume registration is one of the enabling technologies for computer-aided image guidance, bringing high-resolution pre-operative data into the operating room to provide more realistic information about the patient's anatomy [17]. This technique has been used when dealing with several scenarios such as liver surgery [1], radio-frequency thermal ablation of prostate cancer [5], minimally invasive cardiac procedures [12], among many others.

The second problem is the correction of slicewise motion in volumetric acquisitions. In a variety of situations, inter slice motion may appear when capturing a volumetric image. For example, in case of fetal brain imaging (essential to understand neurodevelopmental disabilities in childhood and infancy) [21], fetus motion generates inconsistencies due to the slice acquisition time. Another case is related to functional magnetic resonance images (fMRI), usually acquired as time series of multislice single-shot echoplanar images (EPI). Patient head motion during the experiments may introduce artifacts on activation signal analysis. Slice-to-volume registration can be used to alleviate this problem by registering every slice to an anatomical volumetric reference following the well-know map-slice-to-volume (MSV) method [13].

1.2   Previous Work

Graph-based image registration, where the task is conceived as a discrete labeling problem on a graph, constitutes one of the most efficient and accurate state-of-the-art methods for image registration [22]. Even if they have shown to be particularly suitable to estimate deformable non-linear transformations [10,11], they were also adapted to the linear case [27]. Most of the publications on the field focus on registering images which are in dimensional correspondence (2D/2D or 3D/3D). In case of projective 2D/3D image registration, only linear transformations were estimated using discrete methods by [26,27]. More recently, several graph-based approaches to perform deformable slice-to-volume registration were introduced in [6–8]. In these works, rigid transformations were computed as a by-product of the deformable parameters, leading to unnecessary computational burden (since rigid transformations are by far lower dimensional than deformable ones). To the best of our knowledge, rigid (only) slice-to-volume registration has not been formulated within this powerful framework. To date, all the methods focusing on this challenging problem are based on continuous (e.g. simplex [5], gradient descent [21], Powell's method [9], etc.) or heuristic approaches (evolutionary algorithms [23], simulated annealing [2]), missing the aforementioned advantages offered by discrete optimization. Based on the work of [26], we propose a discrete Markov Random Field (MRF) formulation of this problem, delivering more precise results than the state-of-the-art continuous approaches. Moreover, inspired by the work of [16] in the context of vector flow estimation, we discuss how continuous state-of-the-art approaches can be used to further refine the rigid transformations obtained through discrete optimization, resulting in more accurate solutions.

2   Rigid Slice-to-Volume Registration Through Markov Random Fields

We formulate rigid slice-to-volume registration as an optimization problem. Given a 2D image $I : \Omega_I \in \Re^2 \to \Re$, and a 3D image $J : \Omega_J \in \Re^3 \to \Re$, we aim at recovering the rigid transformation specified by $\pi = (r_x, r_y, r_z, t_x, t_y, t_z)$ that better aligns both images, by solving:

$$\hat{\pi} = \underset{\pi}{\operatorname{argmin}} \, \mathcal{M}(I, \pi[J]), \qquad (1)$$

where $\pi[J]$ corresponds to the slice extracted from image J (using trilinear interpolation) and specified by the rigid transformation π (as explained in Fig. 1). $\mathcal{M}$ is the so-called matching criteria, that quantifies the dissimilarity between the 2D image I and the slice $\pi[J]$. Alternative matching criteria can be adopted depending on the type of images we are registering. For example, in monomodal cases where intensities tend to be linearly correlated in both images, simple functions such as sum of absolute differences (SAD) or sum of squared differences (SSD) may make the job. However, for more complicated cases like multimodal

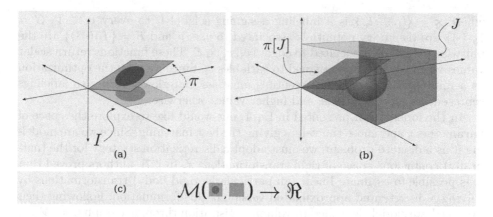

Fig. 1. Interpretation of the components of Eq. 1. (a) Image I corresponds to the input 2D image, which is moved by different rigid transformations π. (b) Image J corresponds to the 3D image. Given a rigid transformation π, a slice $\pi[J]$ is extracted (using trilinear interpolation). In that way, it is possible to explore the space of solutions by sampling several rigid transformations π. (c) The matching criterion $\mathcal{M}$ quantifies the dissimilarity of both 2D images, I and $\pi[J]$. Higher values indicate dissimilar images while lower values indicate better alignment.

registration (where the relation between intensity values in both images is usually non-linear), more elaborated functions like mutual information (MI) are applied.

This optimization problem is commonly solved through continuous (gradient or non-gradient based) methods, which are considerably sensible to initialization and may be stuck in local minima. As discussed in Sect. 1.2, in this work we model rigid slice-to-volume registration as a discrete labeling problem following the discretization strategy proposed by [27].

2.1 Rigid Slice-to-Volume Registration as a Discrete Labeling Problem

Rigid slice-to-volume registration, as well as many other problems in computer vision, can be formulated as a discrete labeling problem on a pairwise Markov Random Field (MRF) [24]. Formally, a discrete pairwise MRF is an undirected graph $\mathcal{G} = \langle \mathcal{V}, \mathcal{E} \rangle$, where each node $v_i \in \mathcal{V}, i = 1...|\mathcal{V}|$ represents a discrete variable. Any two variables v_i, v_j depend on each other if there is an edge $(v_i, v_j) \in \mathcal{E}$ linking the corresponding nodes. The range of values that can be assigned to a discrete variable is determined by the label space L. A discrete labeling problem on a pairwise MRF consists on assigning a label $l_i \in L$ to every $v_i \in \mathcal{V}$, such that the following energy is minimized:

$$\mathcal{P}(\mathbf{x}; G, F) = \sum_{v_i \in V} g_i(l_i) + \sum_{(v_i, v_j) \in \mathcal{E}} f_{ij}(l_i, l_j), \tag{2}$$

where $\mathbf{x} = \{l_1, ..., l_n\}$ is a labeling assigning a label l_i to every $v_i \in \mathcal{V}$, $G = \{g_i(\cdot)\}$ are the unary potentials associated to $v_i \in \mathcal{V}$ and $F = \{f_{ij}(\cdot, \cdot)\}$ are the pairwise potentials associated to edges $(v_i, v_j) \in \mathcal{E}$. These functions return scalar values when labels l_i are assigned to variables v_i. Since we pose the optimization as a minimization problem, potentials must associate lower values to labelings representing good solutions, and higher values otherwise.

In the formulation presented in Eq. 1, one would like to explore the space of parameters π and chose the values giving the best matching. Since we are modeling it as a discrete problem, we must adopt a discretization strategy for the (naturally) continuous space of rigid transformations π. In [27], authors proved that it is possible to estimate linear (an particularly, rigid body) transformations by solving a discrete and approximated version of this formulation. Following their proposal, we model rigid slice-to-volume registration through a graph $\mathcal{G} = \langle \mathcal{V}, \mathcal{E} \rangle$, associating every parameter of the rigid transformation $\pi = (r_x, r_y, r_z, t_x, t_y, t_z)$ to a variable $v_i \in \mathcal{V}$, giving a total of 6 variables (nodes in the graph). $\mathcal{G}$ is a fully connected pairwise graph where $\mathcal{E} = \{(v_i, v_j)\}, \forall i \neq j$, meaning that all variables (parameters) depend on each other. Note that this pairwise model is clearly an approximation, since the real dependency between the parameters is not pairwise but high-order. However, as stated in [27], similar approximations have shown to be good enough to estimate linear transformations, while making the problem tractable.

In our discrete strategy, every parameter v_i is updated through a discrete variation d_{l_i} associated to the label l_i. Given an initial transformation $\pi_0 = (r_x^0, r_y^0, r_z^0, t_x^0, t_y^0, t_z^0)$, we explore the space of solutions by sampling discrete variations of π_0, and choosing the one that generates the slice $\pi[J]$ best matching image I. Therefore, for a maximum size ω_i and a quantization factor κ_i, we consider the following variations to the initial estimate of v_i: $\{0, \pm\frac{\omega_i}{\kappa_i}, \pm\frac{2\omega_i}{\kappa_i}, \pm\frac{3\omega_i}{\kappa_i}, ..., \pm\frac{\kappa_i\omega_i}{\kappa_i}\}$. The total number of labels results $|L| = 2\kappa + 1$. Note that 0 is always included since we give the possibility of keeping the current parameter estimate. For example, in case that v_0 corresponds to r_x, $\omega_0 = 0.2$ and $\kappa_0 = 2$, the label space of v_0 will correspond to $\{r_x^0, r_x^0 \pm 0.1, r_x^0 \pm 0.2\}$.

Ideally, we would like to explore the complete search space around π_0 given by all possible combinations of labels. Since we have an exponential number of potential solutions, we adopt a pairwise approximation where only variations for pairs of variables are considered. This variations are encoded in the pairwise terms of the energy defined in Eq. 2 as $f_{ij}(l_i, l_j) = \mathcal{M}(I, \pi_{l_i, l_j}[J])$. Here π_{l_i, l_j} denotes the updated version of π_0, where only v_i and v_j were modified according to the labels l_i and l_j, while the rest of the parameters remained fixed. Unary potentials g_i are not considered since we are only interested in the interaction between variables. Therefore, the discrete version of the optimization problem introduced in Eq. 1 becomes:

$$\hat{\mathbf{x}} = \underset{\mathbf{x}}{\mathrm{argmin}}\, \mathcal{P}(\mathbf{x}; F) = \underset{\mathbf{x}}{\mathrm{argmin}} \sum_{(v_i, v_j) \in \mathcal{E}} \mathcal{M}(I, \pi_{l_i, l_j}[J]), \qquad (3)$$

where the optimal labeling $\hat{\mathbf{x}}$ represents the final rigid transformation $\hat{\pi}$ used to extract the solution slice $\hat{\pi}[J]$.

2.2 Discrete Optimization

We solve the discrete multi-labeling problem from Eq. 3 using FastPD. FastPD is a discrete optimization algorithm based on principles from linear programming and primal dual strategies, which at the same time generalizes the well known α-expansion [15]. One of the main advantages of FastPD is its modularity/scalability, since it deals with a much wider class of problems than α-expansion, being an order of magnitude faster while providing the same optimality guarantees when performing metric labeling [14]. Our problem does not fulfill the conditions to be considered a metric labeling problem (we refer the reader to [4] for a complete discussion about metric labeling); however, FastPD has shown promising results for similar formulations [27].

FastPD solves a series of max-flow min-cut [3] problems on a graph. In that sense, it is similar to α-expansion which also performs discrete inference on multi-label problems by solving successive binary max-flow min-cut problems. The main difference between these approaches is the construction of the graph where max-flow min-cut algorithm is applied. α-expansion constructs the binary problem by restricting the label space, so that the only options for a given variable are to remain in its current assignment, or to take a label α (which varies in every iteration). Instead, FastPD constructs these binary problems by performing a Linear Programming Relaxation (LPR) of the integer program that represents the discrete MRF formulation.

2.3 Incremental Approach

Discrete approximations of continuous spaces usually suffer from low accuracy (since it is bounded by the quality of the discretization). Thus, we adopt an incremental approach to explore the space of solutions in a finer way. The idea is to successively solve the problem from Eq. 3, using the solution from time t as initialization for time $t + 1$, keeping a fixed number of labels but decreasing the maximum sizes ω_i in a factor α_i. Moreover, we also adopt a pyramidal approach, where we generate a Gaussian pyramid for both input images I and J, and we run the complete incremental approach on every level of the pyramid. In that way, we increase the capture range of our method.

2.4 Simplex Refinement Step

Let us advance one of the conclusions of this work, so that we can motivate the last step of our approach. In Sect. 3.1, we compare the performance of our discrete approach with a continuous method based on simplex [18] algorithm. As we will see, when the initialization π_0 is good enough, both continuous and discrete approaches perform well. In fact, in some cases, simplex is delivering more accurate solutions than discrete. However, as we move away from the initialization, discrete optimization gives more and more significant improvements, thanks to its wider capture range. In order to improve the accuracy of our proposal, and inspired by similar conclusions discussed by [16] in the context of vector flow

Ground Truth (GT)	GT - Initial	GT - Continuous	GT - Discrete	GT - Refined

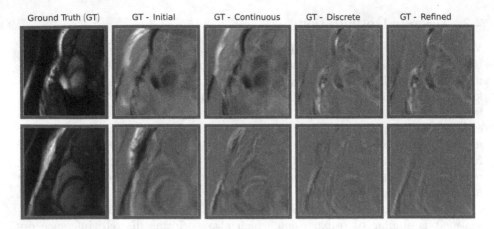

Fig. 2. Visual results for two slices of the individual tests. The first column corresponds to the input 2D slice. The second column shows the difference between the input 2D slice and the initial slice. The other columns show the difference between the input and the one resulting slices applying simplex, discrete and refined approaches. Grey values indicate no difference, while white and black value indicate inconsistencies. As it can be observed, the solution given by the refined approach is outperforming the others.

estimation, we refine the results obtained with our approach by optimizing Eq. 1 through simplex, using the discrete solution as initialization.

3   Experiments and Results

In this section, we present the results obtained using the proposed method (considering also the refined version), and we compare them with a state-of-the-art approach based on continuous optimization trough downhill simplex [18] (also known as Nelder-Mead or amoeba method). Simplex is one of the most popular optimization algorithms used to deal with rigid slice-to-volume registration (some examples are [2,13,20,25]). It is a continuous and derivative-free method, which relies on the notion of simplex (which is a special polytope of $n+1$ vertices living in a n-dimensional space) to explore the space of solutions in a systematic way. We used a dataset composed of MRI images of a beating heart. Given an initial sequence of 3D images $M_i, i = 0..19$ of a beating heart (with a resolution of $192 \times 192 \times 11$ voxels and a voxel size of $1.25 \times 1.25 \times 8$ mm), we generated slices which were used for two different experiments.

3.1   Implementation Details and Parameters Setting

We implemented the three versions of the algorithms discussed in this paper (simplex, discrete and refined) mainly using Python and ITK for image manipulation[1]. For simplex optimization we used the method implemented

---

[1] The source code can be downloaded from https://gitlab.com/franco.stramana1/slice-to-volume.

in *scipy.optimize* package, while discrete optimization was performed using a Python wrapped version of the standard C++ implementation of FastPD. In all the experiments, we used a pyramidal approach with 4 Gaussian levels (3D images where not downsampled in z axis because of the low resolution of the images in this direction). The matching criterion adopted in all the experiments was the sum of squared differences, since pixel intensities are equivalent in both 2D and 3D images. The matching criterion $\mathcal{M}$ based on SSD is simply defined as:

$$\mathcal{M}(I_1, I_2) = \sum_{i \in \Omega} (I_1(i) - I_2(i))^2, \tag{4}$$

For the discrete case, at every pyramid level we decreased the maximum label size for both, rotation ($\omega_{rot} = [0.02, 0.015, 0.0125, 0.01]$rad) and translation ($\omega_{trans} = [7, 6.5, 6, 5]$ mm) parameters. Starting from these maximum sizes, we solved Eq. 3 running FastPD several times per level until no improvement is produced or a maximum number of iterations is achieved ($[200, 100, 150, 600]$), using different label space decreasing factors at every pyramid level ($\alpha = [0.08, 0.07, 0.05, 0.03]$). The total number of labels was fixed to 5 ($\kappa = 2$) for all the experiments. For the continuous case (where Eq. 1 was optimized using simplex), we used again a 4-levels pyramidal approach, with simplex running until convergence in every level. Finally, for the refined experiment, we just ran the simplex experiment initialized with the solution estimated with the discrete method. For every registration case, continuous approach took around 30secs while the discrete version took 9mins, running on a laptop with an Intel i7-4720HQ and 16 GB of RAM.

3.2 Experiments

We performed two different type of experiments, considering individual registration cases as well as image series. For validation, we measured three different indicators: the distance in terms of translation and rotation parameters between the estimated and ground truth transformations, together with the mean of absolute differences (MAD) between the input 2D image and the slice specified by the estimated rigid transformation.

Individual tests. The first set of experiments measures the accuracy of the three approaches using individual tests, where 100 random slices extracted from the 20 volumes are considered as single images (independently of the series), and registered to the first volume M_0. We run the same experiment for every slice using three different initializations (resulting in 300 registration cases), where ground truth parameters were randomly perturbed in three different ranges ($[5, 12), [12, 18), [18, 25)$ millimeters for translation and $[0.1, 0.2), [0.2, 0.3), [0.3, 0.4)$ radians for rotation parameters) to guarantee that both, good and bad initializations, are considered for every slice. Quantitative results are reported in

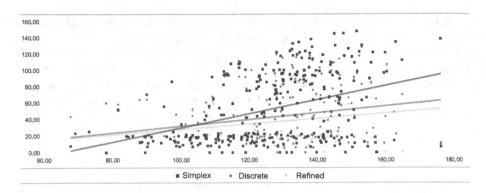

Fig. 3. Individual tests where 100 2D slices (extracted at locations specified using random rigid transformations) are considered as independent registration cases. Every point form the scatter plot represents the mean of absolute differences (MAD) between the input 2D image and the slice extracted at the initial position (X axis) vs the estimated position (Y axis). We also include a linear trend estimation (fitted using least squares method) to compare the robustness of the method to bad initializations.

Table 1. Average error estimated in terms of rotation (expressed in radians), translation (expressed in millimeters) and MAD for the three alternative approaches discussed in this paper. As it can be observed, the discrete and refined methods outperform the standard continuous approach optimized through simplex.

Method	R_x	R_y	R_z	T_x	T_y	T_z	MAD
Simplex	0,14	0,13	0,12	8,46	9,62	10,69	51,88
Discrete	0,12	0,08	0,09	5,87	6,72	6,18	42,36
Refined	**0,10**	**0,07**	**0,08**	**5,09**	**5,96**	**4,92**	**36,45**

Figs. 3 and 4 and summarized in Table 1. Visual results for qualitative evaluation are reported in Fig. 2.

Results in the scatter plot from Fig. 3 indicate that, as we go farther away from the initialization (in this case, it is quantified by the MAD between the input 2D image and the slice corresponding to the initialization), discrete and refined methods tend to be more robust. This robustness is clearly reflected by the slope of the trend lines: the refined method presents the trend line with the lower slope, meaning that even for bad initializations it converges to better solutions. The boxplot from Fig. 4 and the numerical results from Table 1 confirm that discrete and refined methods perform better not only in terms of MAD, but also with respect to the distance between the rotation/translation estimated and ground truth parameters.

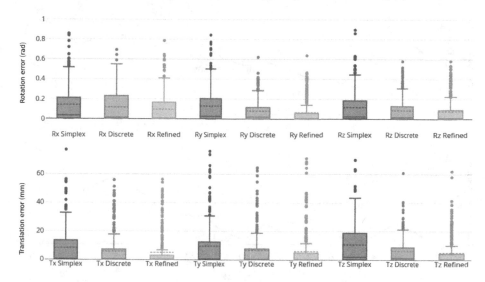

Fig. 4. Boxplot corresponding to the estimated error (in terms of rotation and translation parameters) for the 300 individual tests. As it can be observed, discrete and refined approaches are reducing both the mean error (shown as a dotted line in every box) and the dispersion.

Temporal series test. The idea behind the second experiment is to simulate an image guided surgery (IGS) scenario, where a fixed pre-operative volume must be fused with consecutive intra-operative 2D images suffering deformations (in this case, due to heart beating). Given the temporal sequence of 20 volumetric MRI images $M_i, i = 0..19$, we generated a sequence of 20 2D slices to validate our method. It was extracted as in [8]: starting from a random initial translation $T_0 = (T_{x_0}, T_{y_0}, T_{z_0})$ and rotation $R_0 = (R_{x_0}, R_{y_0}, R_{z_0})$, we extracted a 2D slice I_0 from the initial volume M_0. Gaussian noise was added to every parameter in order to generate the position used to extract the next slice from the next volume. We used $\sigma_r = 3°$ for the rotation and $\sigma_t = 5mm$ for the translation parameters. All the slices were registered to the first volume M_0. The solution of the registration problem for slice I_i was used as initialization for the slice I_{i+1}. The first experiment was initialized randomly perturbing its ground truth transformation with the same noise parameters. As it can be observed in Fig. 5, discrete and refined approaches manage to keep a good estimation error while simplex can not. Note that different strategies could be used in real scenarios to obtain good initializations for the first slice. For example, in IGS, physicians could start from a plane showing always the same anatomical structure, or identify landmark correspondences in the first slice and the 3D image useful to estimate an initial transformation.

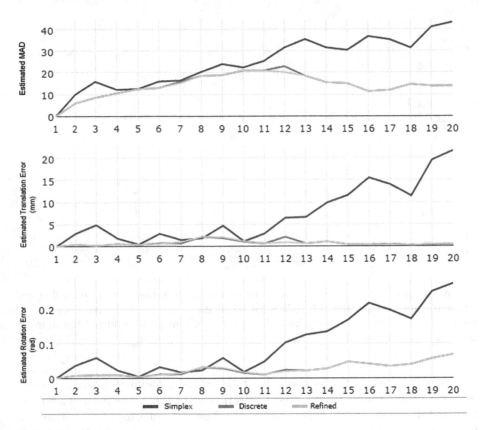

Fig. 5. Results for the temporal series experiment. In this case, the transformation estimated for the slice i was used as initialization for the next slice of the series. We reported results in terms of MAD and rotation/translation error for the estimated transformations using the three approaches.

4   Discussion, Conclusions and Future Works

In this paper we presented a strategy to solve rigid slice-to-volume registration as a discrete graph labeling problem, following the discretization strategy introduced by [27]. We validated our proposal using a MRI dataset of a beating heart, where arbitrary 2D slices are fused with a 3D volume. The experimental results showed that our discrete approach produces more accurate and robust estimates for the rigid transformations than a continuous method based on simplex. Moreover, they also reflected that results obtained using such a method can be further refined using a continuous approach like simplex, leading to even more accurate estimations. This is coherent with the conclusions presented by [16] for the case of optical flow estimation.

An interesting discussion about the limitations of our approach, emerges when we observe the results obtained in previous work by [6–8] using similar images. In these works, both rigid and local deformable parameters are estimated in a one-shot discrete optimization procedure, delivering results which are considerably better than ours, even for the refined approach. Since we are dealing with 2D images which are deformed with respect to the static 3D volume (due to heart beating), estimating both rigid and deformable parameters at the same time seems to be the correct solution since there is a clear mutual dependence between them. However, if we look at the results corresponding to the first slices of the temporal series in Fig. 5 (where there is almost no deformation, and even null deformation for the 1st slice), we can see that the quality of the solution is significantly better than in the other cases. In fact, the error is almost 0. It suggests that when the 2D image is not deformed with respect to the input volume, our method is enough to capture slice-to-volume mapping. This limitation is somehow inherent to the model we are using: rigid transformations can not deal with local deformations. To improve the results in these cases, we plan to extend our approach to linear transformations where also anisotropic scaling and shearing can be considered. Following the strategy by [27], it will result straightforward.

Finally, a future line of research has to do with applying discrete rigid (or linear) slice-to-volume registration to other problems. As discussed in Sect. 1.1 motion correction for volume reconstruction is another problem requiring mapping slice-to-volume. It would be interesting to explore how our approaches performs in this case.

References

1. Bao, P., Warmath, J., Galloway, R., Herline, A.: Ultrasound-to-computer-tomography registration for image-guided laparoscopic liver surgery. Surg. Endosc. **19**, 424–429 (2005)
2. Birkfellner, W., Figl, M., Kettenbach, J., Hummel, J., Homolka, P., Schernthaner, R., Nau, T., Bergmann, H.: Rigid 2D/3D slice-to-volume registration and its application on fluoroscopic CT images. Med. Phys. **34**(1), 246 (2007)
3. Boykov, Y., Kolmogorov, V.: An experimental comparison of min-cut/max- flow algorithms for energy minimization in vision. IEEE TPAMI **26**(9), 1124–1137 (2004)
4. Boykov, Y., Veksler, O., Zabih, R.: Fast approximate energy minimization via graph cuts. IEEE Trans. Pattern Anal. Mach. Intell. **23**(11), 1222–1239 (2001)
5. Fei, B., Duerk, J.L., Boll, D.T., Lewin, J.S., Wilson, D.L.: Slice-to-volume registration and its potential application to interventional MRI-guided radio-frequency thermal ablation of prostate cancer. IEEE Trans. Med. Imaging **22**(4), 515–525 (2003)
6. Ferrante, E., Fecamp, V., Paragios, N.: Implicit planar and in-plane deformable mapping in medical images through high order graphs. In: ISBI 2015, pp. 721–724, April 2015. http://ieeexplore.ieee.org/lpdocs/epic03/wrapper.htm?arnumber=7163974
7. Ferrante, E., Fecamp, V., Paragios, N.: Slice-to-volume deformable registration: efficient one-shot consensus between plane selection and in-plane deformation. IJCARS **10**, 791–800 (2015)

8. Ferrante, Enzo, Paragios, Nikos: Non-rigid 2D-3D medical image registration using markov random fields. In: Mori, Kensaku, Sakuma, Ichiro, Sato, Yoshinobu, Barillot, Christian, Navab, Nassir (eds.) MICCAI 2013. LNCS, vol. 8151, pp. 163–170. Springer, Heidelberg (2013). doi:10.1007/978-3-642-40760-4_21

9. Gholipour, A., Estroff, J.A., Warfield, S.K.: Robust super-resolution volume reconstruction from slice acquisitions: application to fetal brain MRI. IEEE TMI **29**(10), October 2010. http://www.pubmedcentral.nih.gov/articlerender.fcgi? artid=3694441&tool=pmcentrez&rendertype=abstract,   http://ieeexplore.ieee. org/lpdocs/epic03/wrapper.htm?arnumber=5482022

10. Glocker, B., Sotiras, A.: Deformable medical image registration: setting the state of the art with discrete methods. Annu. Rev. Biomed. Eng. **13**, 219–244 (2011)

11. Heinrich, M.P., Jenkinson, M., Brady, M., Schnabel, J.A.: MRF-based deformable registration and ventilation estimation of lung CT. IEEE TMI **32**(7), 1239–1248 (2013)

12. Huang, X., Moore, J., Guiraudon, G., Jones, D.L., Bainbridge, D., Ren, J., Peters, T.M.: Dynamic 2D ultrasound and 3D CT image registration of the beating heart. IEEE TMI **28**(8), 1179–1189 (2009)

13. Kim, B., Boes, J.L., Bland, P.H., Chenevert, T.L., Meyer, C.R.: Motion correction in fMRI via registration of individual slices into an anatomical volume. Magn. Reson. Med. **41**(5), 964–972 (1999)

14. Komodakis, N., Tziritas, G., Paragios, N.: Fast, approximately optimal solutions for single and dynamic MRFs. In: CVPR (2007)

15. Komodakis, N., Tziritas, G., Paragios, N.: Performance vs computational efficiency for optimizing single and dynamic MRFs: setting the state of the art with primal-dual strategies. Comput. Vis. Image Underst. **112**(1), 14–29 (2008). http://linkinghub.elsevier.com/retrieve/pii/S1077314208000982

16. Lempitsky, V., Roth, S., Rother, C.: FusionFlow: discrete-continuous optimization for optical flow estimation. In: CVPR, pp. 1–22 (2008)

17. Liao, R., Zhang, L., Sun, Y., Miao, S., Chefd'Hotel, C.: A review of recent advances in registration techniques applied to minimally invasive therapy. IEEE TMM **15**(5), 983–1000 (2013)

18. Nelder, J.A., Mead, R.: A simplex method for function minimization. Comput. J. **7**(4), 308–313 (1965). http://comjnl.oxfordjournals.org/cgi/doi/10.1093/comjnl/ 7.4.308

19. Paragios, N., Ferrante, E., Glocker, B., Komodakis, N., Parisot, S., Zacharaki, E.I.: (Hyper)-graphical models in biomedical image analysis. Med. Image Anal. (2016). http://linkinghub.elsevier.com/retrieve/pii/S1361841516301062

20. Park, H., Meyer, C.R., Kim, B.: Improved motion correction in fMRI by Joint mapping of slices into an anatomical volume. In: MICCAI, pp. 745–751 (2004)

21. Rousseau, F., Glenn, O.: A novel approach to high resolution fetal brain MR imaging. Medical Image Computing and Computer-Assisted Intervention (MICCAI), vol. 3749, pp. 548–555 (2005). http://link.springer.com/10.1007/11566465

22. Sotiras, A., Davatazikos, C., Paragios, N.: Deformable medical image registration: a survey. IEEE Trans. Med. Imaging **32**, 1153–1190 (2013)

23. Tadayyon, H., Lasso, A., Kaushal, A., Guion, P., Fichtinger, G.: Target motion tracking in MRI-guided transrectal robotic prostate biopsy. IEEE TBE **58**(11), 3135–3142 (2011)

24. Wang, C., Komodakis, N., Paragios, N.: Markov random field modeling, inference & learning in computer vision & image understanding: a survey. CVIU **117**(11), 1610–1627 (2013). http://linkinghub.elsevier.com/retrieve/pii/S1077314213001343

25. Xu, R., Athavale, P., Nachman, A., Wright, G.A.: Multiscale registration of real-time and prior MRI data for image-guided cardiac interventions. IEEE TBE **61**, 2621–2632 (2014)
26. Zikic, D., Glocker, B., Kutter, O., Groher, M., Komodakis, N., Khamene, A., Paragios, N., Navab, N.: Markov random field optimization for intensity-based 2D–3D registration. In: SPIE Medical Imaging, p. 762334. International Society for Optics and Photonics (2010)
27. Zikic, D., Glocker, B., Kutter, O., Groher, M., Komodakis, N., Kamen, A., Paragios, N., Navab, N.: Linear intensity-based image registration by Markov random fields and discrete optimization. Med. Image Anal. **14**(4), 550–562 (2010)

Sparse Probabilistic Parallel Factor Analysis for the Modeling of PET and Task-fMRI Data

Vincent Beliveau[1,2(✉)], Georgios Papoutsakis[3], Jesper Løve Hinrich[3], and Morten Mørup[3]

[1] Faculty of Health and Medical Sciences, University of Copenhagen, Copenhagen, Denmark
[2] Neurobiology Research Unit, Rigshospitalet, Copenhagen, Denmark
vincent.beliveau@nru.dk
[3] DTU Compute, Technical University of Denmark, Copenhagen, Denmark

Abstract. Modern datasets are often multiway in nature and can contain patterns common to a mode of the data (e.g. space, time, and subjects). Multiway decomposition such as parallel factor analysis (PARAFAC) take into account the intrinsic structure of the data, and sparse versions of these methods improve interpretability of the results. Here we propose a variational Bayesian parallel factor analysis (VB-PARAFAC) model and an extension with sparse priors (SP-PARAFAC). Notably, our formulation admits time and subject specific noise modeling as well as subject specific offsets (i.e., mean values). We confirmed the validity of the models through simulation and performed exploratory analysis of positron emission tomography (PET) and functional magnetic resonance imaging (fMRI) data. Although more constrained, the proposed models performed similarly to more flexible models in approximating the PET data, which supports its robustness against noise. For fMRI, both models correctly identified task-related components, but were not able to segregate overlapping activations.

1 Introduction

One of the most widely used tool for dimensionality reduction of large datasets is the Principal Component Analysis (PCA) [1], as well as its probabilistic formulation (PPCA) [2]. PCA finds orthogonal components describing the directions of maximum variance. Selecting the number of components to retain can be problematic and usually requires a post-processing step if the number is not known beforehand. Furthermore, even components explaining a large portion of the variance can include small, non-informative weights making them difficult to interpret. Sparse versions of the PCA algorithms deal with these issues by pruning whole components or individual weights [3].

Neuroscience data are multi-modal in nature and although PCA can be performed on data concatenated along one mode (e.g. time) to identify (e.g. spatial) components common to another mode (e.g. subjects), this approach discards

J.L. Hinrich and M. Mørup were supported by the Lundbeck Foundation (grant. no. R105-9813).

H. Müller et al. (Eds.): MCV/BAMBI 2016, LNCS 10081, pp. 186–198, 2017.
DOI: 10.1007/978-3-319-61188-4_17

mode-specific information (e.g. subject specific scaling). Instead using a multiway decomposition method, such as Parallel Factor Analysis (PARAFAC) also called Canonical Decomposition or Canonical Polyadic Decomposition (CP) [4–6], maintains the intrinsic structure of the data while having substantially less degrees of freedom and thereby being less sensitive to noise, given model assumptions are met. Furthermore, the PARAFAC model is unique (up to scaling and permutation) under mild conditions [7] providing a more interpretable representation, as components cannot be arbitrarily rotated. Exploiting these properties, the PARAFAC model has successfully been applied to the modeling of neuroimaging data such as EEG and fMRI (for reviews see also [8–10]). Similar to PCA, the amount of small non-informative weights can minimized by inducing sparsity on individual weights. A sparse PARAFAC based on least-squares optimization was discussed in [11].

Sparse multiway models have a high relevance in fields such as neuroscience. The brain has been demonstrated to be organized in networks, and for some specific tasks, e.g. motor tasks, distinct regions of the brain are active, hence a spatially sparse pattern can be expected. When this type of task is performed across multiple subjects it is possible to leverage the intrinsic structure of the data by performing multiway decomposition.

In this paper, we develop a fully bayesian sparse probabilistic PARAFAC (SP-PARAFAC) model with time-dependent and subject specific isotropic noise. We show how a simple change to the sparsity prior allows for easy transition between SP-PARAFAC and probabilistic PARAFAC (VB-PARAFAC). Approximate solution are given based on variational Bayesian inference [12] and we investigate the applicability of the models to PET and task-based fMRI data. While probabilistic PARAFAC has previously been investigated (cf. [13–16]) none impose sparsity on individual elements nor model time-dependent noise.

2 Review of Probabilistic PCA

The initial formulation of probabilistic PCA [2] defines a model relating observations x to latent variables z projected on a K dimensional hyperplane W of origin m with additive Gaussian noise ϵ, such that $x = Wz + m + \epsilon$. Here, the latent variable and the noise are assumed to follow an isotropic Gaussian: $z \sim \mathcal{N}(0, I)$ and $\epsilon \sim \mathcal{N}(0, \tau^{-1}I)$, where τ is the precision of the noise.

In subsequent work [17], the authors formulated a fully Bayesian treatment of PCA solved through variational inference (VB-PCA) and with hierarchical ARD priors $P(W|\alpha)$ over the columns of the matrix W, allowing for automatic selection of the number of components. Here $P(W|\alpha)$ was defined to follow a multivariate Gaussian specific to each column where α is defined as the precision:

$$P(\boldsymbol{W}|\boldsymbol{\alpha}) = \prod_k^K \left(\frac{\alpha_k}{2\pi}\right)^{\frac{T}{2}} \exp\left\{-\frac{1}{2}\alpha_k\|\boldsymbol{w}_k\|^2\right\} \tag{1}$$

$$P(\boldsymbol{\alpha}) = \prod_k^K \Gamma(\alpha_k|a_{\alpha_k}, b_{\alpha_k}) \tag{2}$$

where $\boldsymbol{w}_k$ is the k_{th} column of $\boldsymbol{W}$. To complete the Bayesian specification, the remaining parameters are associated with broad priors: $\boldsymbol{m} \sim \mathcal{N}(0, \beta^{-1}\boldsymbol{I})$ and $\tau \sim \Gamma(a_\tau, b_\tau)$.

The investigation of alternative priors on $\boldsymbol{W}$ by [3] lead to the a fully sparse formulation of PCA (SP-PCA) where a sparsity inducing prior is imposed on elements of $\boldsymbol{W}$ rather than columns. In theory this allows the model to identify both the model order (true K) and disregard noisy or irrelevant voxels (features). Among the different priors studied, Jeffrey's prior was shown to give sparse components with the highest cumulative explained variance. With Jeffrey's prior, the conditional distribution of $P(\boldsymbol{W}|\boldsymbol{\alpha})$ and the prior on $\boldsymbol{\alpha}$ becomes:

$$P(w_{v,k}|\alpha_{v,k}) = \left(\frac{\alpha_{v,k}}{2\pi}\right)^{1/2} \exp\left\{-\frac{1}{2}\alpha_{v,k}w_{v,k}^2\right\} \tag{3}$$

$$Jeffrey's(\alpha_{v,k}) \sim \sqrt{E_{P(w_{v,k}|\alpha_{v,k})}\left(\left(\frac{\partial}{\partial\alpha}\ln P(w_{v,k}|\alpha_{v,k})\right)^2\right)} = \frac{1}{\alpha_{v,k}} \tag{4}$$

3   Probabilistic Parallel Factor Analysis

Multiway data can be viewed as a tensor structure. In this paper we are considering 3-way tensors of dimension $V \times T \times S$, where for ease of correspondence with the PET and fMRI datasets V will be referred to as voxels, T as time and S as subjects. Similar to PCA, the PARAFAC model seeks to identify a matrix $\boldsymbol{W}$ of size $V \times K$, for which the columns are common components across the S subjects. In contrast to PCA the PARAFAC model allows for individual scaling of the components, which can be used to characterize inter-subject variability and it also accounts for subject specific temporal noise. A graphical model of the proposed model is illustrated in Fig. 1. Each timepoint t for each subject s is reconstructed by,

$$\boldsymbol{x}_t^{(s)} = \boldsymbol{W}\mathrm{diag}(\boldsymbol{\delta}^{(s)})\boldsymbol{z}_t + \boldsymbol{m}^{(s)} + \boldsymbol{\epsilon}_t^{(s)} \tag{5}$$

where $\boldsymbol{W}$ and $\boldsymbol{z}$ are now common across subjects, but where we model time dependent noise specific to each subject $\boldsymbol{\epsilon}_t^{(s)}$ (with precision $\tau_t^{(s)}$), subject specific mean $\boldsymbol{m}^{(s)}$ and subject specific scaling of the components $\boldsymbol{\delta}^{(s)}$. Note that here $\boldsymbol{\epsilon}$, $\boldsymbol{m}$, $\boldsymbol{\delta}$ and τ are matrices and $\cdot^{(s)}$ denotes the sth column. The likelihood of a model with a given set of parameters is assess by,

$$P(\boldsymbol{X}|\boldsymbol{W}, \boldsymbol{Z}, \boldsymbol{m}, \tau, \boldsymbol{\delta}) = \prod_s^S \prod_t^T \mathcal{N}\left(\boldsymbol{x}_t^{(s)}|\boldsymbol{W}\mathrm{diag}(\boldsymbol{\delta}^{(s)})\boldsymbol{z}_t + \boldsymbol{m}^{(s)}, \tau_t^{(s)^{-1}}\boldsymbol{I}_V\right) \tag{6}$$

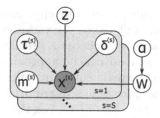

Fig. 1. Graphical model for probabilistic PARAFAC.

To complete the Bayesian framework, prior distributions are defined for the parameters:

$$P(\boldsymbol{\delta}) = \prod_s^S \mathcal{N}\left(\boldsymbol{\delta}^{(s)} | \mathbf{0}, \boldsymbol{I}_K\right) \tag{7}$$

$$P(\boldsymbol{\tau}) = \prod_s^S \prod_t^T \Gamma\left(\tau_t^{(s)} | a_{\tau_t^{(s)}}, b_{\tau_t^{(s)}}\right) \tag{8}$$

$$P(\boldsymbol{m}) = \prod_s^S \mathcal{N}\left(\boldsymbol{m}^{(s)} | \mathbf{0}, \beta^{-1} \boldsymbol{I}_V\right) \tag{9}$$

$$P(\boldsymbol{Z}) = \prod_t^T \mathcal{N}\left(\boldsymbol{z}_t | \mathbf{0}, \boldsymbol{I}_K\right) \tag{10}$$

The choice of priors for $\boldsymbol{W}$ and $\boldsymbol{\alpha}$ determines the pruning and sparsity capability of the model. If the priors are chosen to be Eqs. (1) and (2) then VB-PARAFAC is obtained. Which seeks to identify active and inactive components using ARD. However, if the priors are chosen to be Eqs. (3) and (4) then Sparse Probabilistic (SP-)PARAFAC is obtained. Seeking to identify both dimensionality (model order) and active voxels (features).

The general complexity of the VB- and SP-PCA and the proposed VB- and SP-PARAFAC models differ. Notably, the PCA models with temporally concatenated data have $KT(S-1)$ more degrees of freedom for the latent variable z compared to the PARAFAC models, which for a dataset with large T and K could be a potential source of overfitting, whereas PARAFAC have KS more parameters for $\boldsymbol{\delta}$ and $V(S-1)$ more parameters for $\boldsymbol{m}$.

4   Variational Inference

In order to maximize the likelihood function the marginal distribution $P(\boldsymbol{X}) = \int P(\boldsymbol{X}, \theta) d\theta$ must be estimated. However, the marginalization of this distribution with respect to the prior distributions is most often analytically intractable.

Variational inference solves this problem by approximating the desired distribution with another distribution Q, called the variational distribution. The challenge in a variational approach is to choose a sufficiently simple distribution Q so that the log marginal likelihood can be approximated by a tractable lower bound $\mathcal{L}(Q)$ and at the same time is sufficiently flexible in order to make this bound tight. A common choice for Q is a distribution which factorizes over the model parameters such that $Q = \prod_i Q_i(\theta_i)$. For the VB-PARAFAC model, the distribution $Q_i(\theta_i)$ were defined as follow:

$$Q(\mathbf{Z}) = \prod_t^T \mathcal{N}(\boldsymbol{\mu}_{\mathbf{z}_t}, \boldsymbol{\Sigma}_{\mathbf{z}_t}) \tag{11}$$

$$Q(\mathbf{W}) = \prod_v^V \mathcal{N}(\boldsymbol{w}_v | \boldsymbol{\mu}_{\boldsymbol{w}_v}, \boldsymbol{\Sigma}_{\boldsymbol{w}_v}) \tag{12}$$

$$Q(\boldsymbol{\alpha}) = \prod_k^K \Gamma(\alpha_k | \tilde{a}_{\alpha_k}, \tilde{b}_{\alpha_k}) \tag{13}$$

$$Q(\boldsymbol{\delta}) = \prod_s^S \mathcal{N}(\boldsymbol{\delta}^{(s)} | \boldsymbol{\mu}_{\boldsymbol{\delta}^{(s)}}, \boldsymbol{\Sigma}_{\boldsymbol{\delta}^{(s)}}) \tag{14}$$

$$Q(\boldsymbol{m}) = \prod_s^S \mathcal{N}(\boldsymbol{m}^{(s)} | \boldsymbol{\mu}_{\boldsymbol{m}^{(s)}}, \boldsymbol{\Sigma}_{\boldsymbol{m}^{(s)}}) \tag{15}$$

$$Q(\boldsymbol{\tau}) = \prod_s^S \prod_t^T \Gamma(\tau_t^{(s)} | \tilde{a}_{\tau_t^{(s)}}, \tilde{s}_{\tau_t^{(s)}}) \tag{16}$$

It can be shown that the log marginal probability is equivalent to $\ln P(X) = \mathcal{L}(Q) + KL(Q \| P)$, where KL is the Kullback-Leibler divergence. By fixing Q_j and maximizing $\mathcal{L}(Q)$ with respect to the remaining $Q_{i \neq j}$ we obtain the general expression $\ln Q_j^* = \mathbb{E}_{i \neq j}[\ln p(\mathbf{X}, \boldsymbol{\theta})] + const$ which minimizes the KL divergence. By applying and normalizing this, the update rules for Q can be derived and are shown in Eqs. 17 – 27. Note that $\boldsymbol{w}_v$ denotes a row of $\mathbf{W}$, $\langle \cdot \rangle$ denotes the expectation and that the operator $\bullet$ is the Hadamard product.

$$\boldsymbol{\mu}_{\boldsymbol{\delta}^{(s)}} = \boldsymbol{\Sigma}_{\boldsymbol{\delta}^{(s)}} \sum_t^T \left\langle \tau_t^{(s)} \right\rangle \langle \mathrm{diag}(\boldsymbol{z}_t) \rangle \left\langle \mathbf{W}^T \right\rangle (\boldsymbol{x}_t^{(s)} - \left\langle \boldsymbol{m}^{(s)} \right\rangle) \tag{17}$$

$$\boldsymbol{\Sigma}_{\boldsymbol{\delta}^{(s)}} = \left(\mathbf{I}_K + \sum_t^T \left\langle \tau_t^{(s)} \right\rangle \langle \boldsymbol{z}_t \boldsymbol{z}_t^T \rangle \bullet \langle \mathbf{W}^T \mathbf{W} \rangle \right)^{-1} \tag{18}$$

$$\boldsymbol{\mu}_{\boldsymbol{z}_t} = \boldsymbol{\Sigma}_{\boldsymbol{z}_t} \sum_s^S \left\langle \tau_t^{(s)} \right\rangle \mathrm{diag}\left(\left\langle \boldsymbol{\delta}^{(s)} \right\rangle \right) \left\langle \mathbf{W}^T \right\rangle \left(\boldsymbol{x}_t^{(s)} - \left\langle \boldsymbol{m}^{(s)} \right\rangle \right) \tag{19}$$

$$\Sigma_{z_t} = \left(I_K + \sum_s^S \left\langle \tau_t^{(s)} \right\rangle \left\langle \delta^{(s)} \delta^{(s)T} \right\rangle \bullet \left\langle W^T W \right\rangle \right)^{-1} \tag{20}$$

$$\mu_{m^{(s)}} = \Sigma_{m^{(s)}} \sum_t^T \left\langle \tau_t^{(s)} \right\rangle \left(x_t^{(s)} - \langle W \rangle \left\langle diag(\delta^{(s)}) \right\rangle \langle z_t \rangle \right) \tag{21}$$

$$\Sigma_{m^{(s)}} = \left(\beta + \sum_t^T \langle \tau \rangle_t^{(s)} \right)^{-1} I_K \tag{22}$$

$$\mu_{w_v} = \Sigma_{w_v} \sum_s^S \sum_t^T \left\langle diag(\delta^{(s)}) \right\rangle \langle z_t \rangle \left\langle \tau_t^{(s)} \right\rangle \left(x_t^{(s)T} - \left\langle m^{(s)T} \right\rangle \right)_v \tag{23}$$

$$\Sigma_{w_v} = \left(diag(\alpha) + \sum_s^S \sum_t^T \left\langle \tau_t^{(s)} \right\rangle \left\langle \delta^{(s)} \delta^{(s)T} \right\rangle \bullet \left\langle z_t z_t^T \right\rangle \right)^{-1} \tag{24}$$

$$\tilde{a}_\alpha = a_\alpha + \frac{V}{2}, \quad \tilde{b}_{\alpha_k} = b_{\alpha_k} + \frac{\left\langle w_k^T w_k \right\rangle}{2} \tag{25}$$

$$\tilde{a}_{\tau^{(s)}} = a_{\tau^{(s)}} + \frac{V}{2} \tag{26}$$

$$\begin{aligned}
\tilde{b}_{\tau_t^{(s)}} = b_{\tau_t^{(s)}} & + \frac{1}{2} \| x_t^{(s)} \|^2 + \frac{1}{2} \left\langle \| m^{(s)} \|^2 \right\rangle - x_t^{(s)T} \left\langle m^{(s)} \right\rangle \\
& - x_t^{(s)T} \langle W \rangle \left\langle diag(\delta^{(s)}) \right\rangle \langle z_t \rangle \\
& + \frac{1}{2} Tr \left(\langle W^T W \rangle \bullet \left\langle \delta^{(s)} \delta^{(s)T} \right\rangle \langle z_t z_t^T \rangle \right) \\
& + \left\langle m^{(s)T} \right\rangle \langle W \rangle \left\langle diag(\delta^{(s)}) \right\rangle \langle z_t \rangle
\end{aligned} \tag{27}$$

By changing the prior on W to Jeffrey's prior shown in Eq. 4 we obtain the solution for SP-PARAFAC. The Q_i distributions remain the same except for $Q(\alpha)$ which now factorizes over elements, i.e. $Q(\alpha) = \prod_v^V \prod_k^K \Gamma(\alpha_{v,k} | \tilde{a}_{\alpha_{v,k}}, \tilde{b}_{\alpha_{v,k}})$. These changes are reflected in the update rules for W and α,

$$\Sigma_{w_v} = \left(\sum_s^S \sum_t^T \left\langle \tau_t^{(s)} \right\rangle \left\langle \delta^{(s)} \delta^{(s)T} \right\rangle \bullet \left\langle z_t z_t^T \right\rangle + diag(\langle \alpha_{v,\cdot} \rangle) \right)^{-1} \tag{28}$$

$$\tilde{a}_{\alpha_{v,k}} = \frac{1}{2}, \quad \tilde{b}_{\alpha_{v,k}} = \frac{\left\langle w_{v,k}^2 \right\rangle}{2} \tag{29}$$

The lower bound $\mathcal{L}(Q)$ can be easily derived to monitor the convergence of the algorithm. Although convergence is guaranteed, the solution will not necessarily arrive at a global maximum. This is typically addressed by running the algorithm multiple times and keeping the solution with the largest lower bound.

5   Results

In this section, we present a validation of our model with simulation and perform the analysis of PET and fMRI data. The parameters β^{-1}, a_α, b_α, a_τ and b_τ were set to 10^{-3} to obtain broad priors. In all cases, W was initialized using PCA, which in practice consistently lead to a higher lower bound compared to random initialization and mitigated the need for multiple restarts in the case of VB- and SP-PCA. For VB- and SP-PARAFAC, PCA was performed on the data from individual subjects, hence the algorithm was restarted for each subject and the solution with the highest lower bound was kept. To assess stability of the solution across model initializations the RV coefficient [18] between the estimated W for two different initializations was calculated. This was done for all unique pairwise combinations, $(\#repeats-1)!$, and the average RV coefficient is reported. The RV coefficient is a multivariate generalization of the Pearson correlation coefficient which measure subspace overlap and is invariant to rotation and translation. The RV coefficient is one if the subspaces overlap completely and zero if they have no overlap. Similarly, we also computed an average correlation: first, for each pair of estimated W, components were matched based on correlation and an average correlation computed. Then, the average of all unique pairs was computed.

Results were also compared to solutions obtained with the PARAFAC function from the N-way toolbox 3.21 [19], which evaluates the standard PARAFAC model without modeling of the mean or the noise. As PARAFAC does not model the mean, the data was centered when using this algorithm. Due to memory limitation, the PCA initialization for N-way PARAFAC did not work for large datasets, hence we used the default initialization as it consistently resulted in lower reconstruction error compared to random initialization. Furthermore, the number of components was determined by performing the decomposition for a range of varying number of components and keeping the solution with the most components and a core-consistency of a 100.

5.1   Simulation

This section presents a comparison between VB-PCA [17], SP-PCA [3], PARAFAC [20] and the proposed VB-PARAFAC and SP-PARAFAC through simulation. We created a 3-way dataset using the following procedure. Three sparse vectors of length $V = 10$ were created and concatenated to form matrix W; this is shown in Fig. 2 as ground truth. Then random latent variables z_t of length $T = 100$, random mean values $m^{(s)}$ and random scaling factors $\delta^{(s)}$ for $S = 5$ subjects were sampled from the distribution $\mathcal{N}(0, I)$ and linearly mixed according to Eq. 5. The additive noise was sampled from $\mathcal{N}(0, \tau_t^{(s)} I)$, with the precision $\tau_t^{(s)}$ sampled from $\Gamma(1, 1)$. The resulting data was concatenated along the time dimension for the PCA algorithms and as a 3-way tensor for the PARAFAC models.

Figure 2 shows the components identified by the algorithms. All models identified the ground truth components to varying degrees of accuracy and pruned

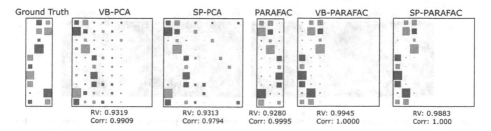

Fig. 2. Hinton diagram of W identified by the algorithms (green is positive and red is negative). Average RV and Pearson's correlation coefficients between the ground truth W and the identified solutions are reported. (Color figure online)

non-informative components. Both PCA models were more confounded by noise and their inability to account for subject specific means compared to their PARAFAC counter parts. Furthermore, SP-PCA and SP-PARAFAC performed better than their VB version at pruning individual non-related weights, although this is not reflected by the RV coefficient. These results indicate that the VB- and SP-PARAFAC models benefit by having PARAFAC structure and by modeling time and subject varying noise as well as subject specific means when these effects are present in the data and that fully sparse priors are more efficient at identifying sparsity structure from the data compared to priors inducing sparsity on whole components.

5.2 Positron Emission Tomography

Here we performed an exploratory data decomposition of PET data. The synchronized nature of PET experiments, the time-depend noise associated with the radioactive isotope decay and subject specific scaling of the time-activity curves (TAC) due to variation in injected dose and body weight make multiway model in theory well suited for the analysis of PET data.

The PET data for the radioligand $[^{11}C]$CUMI-101 and matching T1-weighted structural magnetic resonance images (MRI) were obtained from the Cimbi database [21] for 4 healthy subjects. Dynamic PET images (34 frames; 2×5 s, 10×15 s, 4×30 s, 5×120 s, 5×300 s, 8×600 s) were acquired on a HRRT scanner with approximate in-plane resolution of 2 mm and the structural images were acquired on a 3T Siemens Trio scanner at 1 mm isotropic resolution. The structural images were processed within FreeSurfer [22]. PET images were coregistered to the structural MRI [23], transferred to a common space (MNI152) and smoothed using a 5 mm FWHM 3d Gaussian kernel. The data was finally concatenated along subjects, forming a 3-way tensor, and processed with VB-PARAFAC and SP-PARAFAC with an initial dimensionality of 30.

VB-PCA, VB-PARAFAC and SP-PARAFAC identified 7, 24 and 19 non-null components, respectively; SP-PCA did not prune any component. Only two components were commonly identified by all five methods. The first one loaded on all brain space (Fig. 3A), whereas the second loaded on regions of high and

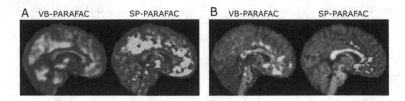

Fig. 3. All algorithms identified at least two similar components, one weighted over the whole brain (A) and one distributed over high and low binding regions (B). Corresponding components for VB-PCA, SP-PCA and PARAFAC are not shown, but exhibited similar patterns. All other components displayed random patterns with no underlying anatomical correspondence. The average RV and Pearson's correlation coefficients for VB- and SP-PARAFAC were (0.5302, 0.5655) and (0.2635, 0.2752).

low binding regions with corresponding weights (Fig. 3B). The others exhibited random patterns across the whole brain and adjusted for small, random variation in the data. There was no component which loaded uniquely on specific brain regions indicating that a set of basis function common to all brain voxel is the more appropriate model. This results is reasonable as the kinetic across all brain voxels is highly similar compared to other modalities, e.g. fMRI. Consequently, although both VB- and SP-PARAFAC algorithms pruned non-informative components, the SP-PARAFAC model introduced seemingly random spatial sparsity which left the components difficult to interpret. Although sparsity is often a desired property, this result indicate that a fully sparse model may not always be appropriate for the identification of global patterns.

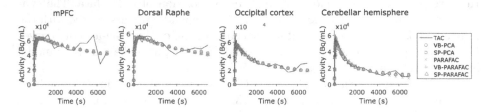

Fig. 4. TACs from individual voxels of selected brain regions and their approximation.

Another interesting application of data decomposition methods applied to PET imaging is the denoising of the data. We compared the approximation performed by the different algorithms and the results were surprisingly similar for all brain regions (see Fig. 4). These results indicate that our constrained PARAFAC models is able to identify noise structure comparable to what a more flexible model like VB and SP-PCA can discover and performed similarly well in approximating the underlying data.

5.3 Functional MRI

The analysis of multiway fMRI data is routinely performed using independent component analysis (ICA) [24]. One of the most common model used to perform ICA decomposition of fMRI data is the probabilistic ICA (PICA) [25] and its tensorial extension for multi-subject analysis. We here aim to demonstrate a side-by-side comparison of the components identified by tensor PICA and the other five methods.

Eight healthy right-handed subjects performed a visually cued reaction fist-closure fMRI task. Subjects performed 10 blocks of a duration of 10 sec, interleaved with 10 sec rest, were they were instructed with a visual cue to open and close their right or left hand at a frequency of approximately 1 Hz; the pattern of left and right blocks was random but fixed across subjects. This task leads to significant activation of the visual, motor and premotor cortex on the contralateral side of the movement, and relatively weaker activation on the ipsilateral side. For each subject, 210 axial echo-planar volumes (TE $= 30$ ms, TR $= 2.25$ s, $64 \times 64 \times 32$ voxels at $3.6 \times 3.6 \times 3.8$ mm) were acquired on a 3-T Siemens Prisma together with a T1-weighted anatomical image at 1 mm isotropic resolution. The fMRI was motion corrected (MCFLIRT [26]), coregistered to the structural image using (FLIRT [26]), transformed to common MNI152 space (FNIRT [20]) and finally smoothed using a 8 mm FWHM 3d Gaussian kernel. The fMRI data was finally processed using tensor PICA in Melodic [25] and the five methods. VB-PARAFAC and SP-PARAFAC had an initial dimensionality of 50. Significance maps were estimated as in [25] by creating Z-scores maps by dividing each components by the residual voxel variance and modeling the associated histograms using a Gaussian/Gamma mixture modeling approach in Melodic.

For PICA, the estimated dimensionality was 47. No component was completely pruned by VB-PARAFAC, whereas SP-PARAFAC identified only 4 components. The components identified by all the models corresponding to motor or visual activation are presented in Fig. 5. The different functional aspect of the task are clearly segregated in the components identified by PICA; component 1 is has strong visual activation (but also contains weaker motor activation), where as components 2 and 3 have strong motor activation corresponding to left and right fist-closure, respectively. For the other methods, all relevant components contained both motor and visual activation, however the significance was relatively lower. This is surprising as we would have expected that by enforcing spatial sparsity and modeling time-dependent noise, which is particularly problematic in fMRI (e.g. physiological artifacts, motion), the identifiability of the signal would have improved. As the activation of the visual and motor areas are synchronized in this task, the visual and motor cortex exhibit similar, but non identical, temporal profile which may be difficult to isolate given our model assumptions. Furthermore, this task also illicits both contralateral and (weaker) ipsilateral activation of the motor and premotor cortex, hence left and right hand squeeze will have overlapping activation which may be difficult to segregate in a sparse model. The SP-PCA and the PARAFAC model clearly underperformed in

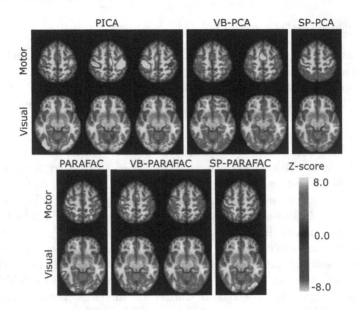

Fig. 5. Motor and visual components (columns) identified by the six methods. The axial slice for the motor and visual views correspond respectively to Z = 55.75 mm and Z = −10.50 mm in MNI152 space. The average RV and Pearson's correlation coefficients for VB- and SP-PARAFAC were (0.9130, 0.6815) and (0.5633, 0.5965).

identifying the motor and visual components. Interestingly, the SP-PARAFAC model was able to prune most of the non task-related components and established a model dimensionality much closer to what is expected from the task compared to the other models.

6   Summary

In this work we presented a VB-PARAFAC model with time-dependent modeling of the noise and a fully sparse extension, the SP-PARAFAC model. We validated these models and compared them to VB-PCA, SP-PCA and PARAFAC through simulation and applied them to PET and task-based fMRI data. For PET, the models identified two common components and performed equally well at approximating the data. The spatial sparsity enforced by SP-PCA and SP-PARAFAC appeared unfortunately random, rendering the components difficult to interpret. We also compared the models to tensor PICA in the identification of task-related fMRI components. Tensor PICA identified functionally segregated motor and visual components where as the other models only identified components with both motor and visual activation and with lower significance. However, the dimensionality of the SP-PARAFAC model was much closer to the what expected given the task, suggesting that this model performs better at pruning non task-related components. Although we solely investigated neuroimaging modalities in this report, these models have a strong relevance for other types of data for which PARAFAC is commonly used.

References

1. Jolliffe, I.: Principal Component Analysis, vol. 487. Springer, New York (1986)
2. Tipping, M., Bishop, C.: Probabilistic principal component analysis. Royal Stat. Soc. **23**(3), 492–503 (1999)
3. Guan, Y., Dy, J.: Sparse probabilistic principal component analysis. In: International Conference on Artificial Intelligence and Statistics, pp. 185–192 (2009)
4. Harshman, R.: Foundations of the parafac procedure: models and conditions for an "explanatory" multi-modal factor analysis. (1970)
5. Carroll, J., Chang, J.: Analysis of individual differences in multidimensional scaling via an n-way generalization of eckart-young decomposition. Psychometrika **35**(3), 283–319 (1970)
6. Hitchcock, F.: The expression of a tensor or a polyadic as a sum of products. J. Math. Phys. **6**(1), 164–189 (1927)
7. Kruskal, J.: Three-way arrays: rank and uniqueness of trilinear decompositions, with application to arithmetic complexity and statistics. Linear Algebra Appl. **18**(2), 95–138 (1977)
8. Kolda, T., Bader, B.: Tensor decompositions and applications. SIAM Rev. **51**(3), 455–500 (2009)
9. Acar, E., Yener, B.: Unsupervised multiway data analysis: a literature survey. IEEE Trans. Knowl. Data Eng. **21**(1), 6–20 (2009)
10. Mørup, M.: Applications of tensor (multiway array) factorizations and decompositions in data mining. Wiley Interdisc. Rev. Data Mining Knowl. Disc. **1**(1), 24–40 (2011)
11. Rasmussen, M., Bro, R.: A tutorial on the lasso approach to sparse modeling. Chemometr. Intell. Lab. Syst. **119**, 21–31 (2012)
12. Attias, H.: A variational bayesian framework for graphical models. Adv. Neural Inform. Process. Syst. **12**(1–2), 209–215 (2000)
13. Nielsen, F.: Variational approach to factor analysis and related models (2004)
14. Ermis, B., Cemgil, A.: A Bayesian tensor factorization model via variational inference for link prediction **3**, 1–9. arXiv preprint arXiv:1409.8276 (2014)
15. Zhao, Q., Zhang, L., Cichocki, A., Hoff, P.: Bayesian CP factorization of incomplete tensors with automatic rank determination **37**(9), 1–15. arXiv preprint arXiv:1401.6497v2 (2015)
16. Guo, W., Yu, W.: Variational Bayesian PARAFAC decomposition for Multidimensional Harmonic Retrieval. In: Proceedings of 2011 IEEE CIE International Conference on Radar, RADAR 2011, vol. 2, pp. 1864–1867 (2011)
17. Bishop, C.: Variational principal components. In: Ninth International Conference on Artificial Neural Networks, ICANN 1999 (Conf. Publ. No. 470), vol. 1, pp. 509–514. IET (1999)
18. Robert, P., Escoufier, Y.: A unifying tool for linear multivariate statistical methods: the RV-coefficient. Appl. Stat. **25**, 257–265 (1976)
19. Andersson, C.A., Bro, R.: The N-way toolbox for MATLAB. Chemometr. Intell. Lab. Syst. **52**(1), 1–4 (2000)
20. Andersson, J., Jenkinson, M., Smith, S.: Non-linear registration aka Spatial normalisation. FMRIB Technial report TR07JA2, p. 22, June 2007

21. Knudsen, G., Jensen, P., Erritzoe, D., Baaré, W., Ettrup, A., Fisher, P., Gillings, N., Hansen, H., Hansen, L., Hasselbalch, S., Henningsson, S., Herth, M., Holst, K., Iversen, P., Kessing, L., Macoveanu, J., Madsen, K., Mortensen, E., Nielsen, F., Paulson, O., Siebner, H., Stenbæk, D., Svarer, C., Jernigan, T., Strother, S., Frokjaer, V.: The center for integrated molecular brain imaging (Cimbi) database. NeuroImage **124**, 1213–1219 (2015)
22. Fischl, B.: FreeSurfer. Neuroimage **62**(2), 774–781 (2012)
23. Greve, D., Fischl, B.: Accurate and robust brain image alignment using boundary-based registration. Neuroimage **48**(1), 63–72 (2009)
24. Calhoun, V., Liu, J., Adali, T.: A review of group ICA for fMRI data and ICA for joint inference of imaging, genetic, and ERP data. NeuroImage **45**(1 Suppl), S163–S172 (2009)
25. Beckmann, C., Smith, S.: Tensorial extensions of independent component analysis for multisubject FMRI analysis. NeuroImage **25**(1), 294–311 (2005)
26. Jenkinson, M., Bannister, P., Brady, M., Smith, S.: Improved optimization for the robust and accurate linear registration and motion correction of brain images. NeuroImage **17**(2), 825–841 (2002)

Non-local Graph-Based Regularization
for Deformable Image Registration

Bartłomiej W. Papież[1(✉)], Adam Szmul[1], Vicente Grau[1], J. Michael Brady[2],
and Julia A. Schnabel[1,3]

[1] Department of Engineering Science, Institute of Biomedical Engineering,
University of Oxford, Oxford, UK
bartlomiej.papiez@eng.ox.ac.uk
[2] Department of Oncology, University of Oxford, Oxford, UK
[3] Division of Imaging Sciences and Biomedical Engineering,
Department of Biomedical Engineering, King's College London, London, UK

Abstract. Deformable image registration aims to deliver a plausible
spatial transformation between two or more images by solving a highly
dimensional, ill-posed optimization problem. Covering the complexity
of physiological motion has so far been limited to either generic physical models or local motion regularization models. This paper presents
an alternative, graphical regularization model, which captures well the
non-local scale of motion, and thus enables to incorporate complex regularization models directly into deformable image registration. In order
to build the proposed graph-based regularization, a Minimum Spanning
Tree (MST), which represents the underlying tissue physiology in a perceptually meaningful way, is computed first. This is followed by a fast
non-local cost aggregation algorithm that performs regularization of the
estimated displacement field using the precomputed MST. To demonstrate the advantage of the presented regularization, we embed it into
the widely used Demons registration framework. The presented method
is shown to improve the accuracy for exhale-inhale CT data pairs.

1 Introduction

Deformable image registration (DIR) algorithms developed for medical imaging applications generally suffer a trade-off between computational complexity
and medical plausibility [1]. From a biomedical standpoint, it is a fundamental
requirement that DIR delivers a geometrical transformation that is *plausible* in
an anatomical, physiological, or functional sense, whichever is appropriate to the
application. From a mathematical standpoint, DIR is a (very) high-dimensional,
ill-posed problem with several millions of degrees of freedom. Many widely-used
regularization models are based on a generic physical model such as diffusion [2],
while more challenging applications may require additional global constraints,
e.g. that the deformation field be a diffeomorphism [3].

Alternatively, in order to accurately model local deformations, a number of
local structure or motion preservation models have been proposed [4–6]. However,
the deformations within or between human organs are often highly complex and

© Springer International Publishing AG 2017
H. Müller et al. (Eds.): MCV/BAMBI 2016, LNCS 10081, pp. 199–207, 2017.
DOI: 10.1007/978-3-319-61188-4_18

do not occur at a single spatial scale. For example, respiratory-induced motion differs for each lung lobe (usually greater in the lower lobes), while the action of the diaphragm and respiratory muscles produces sliding motion at the pleural cavity boundaries. Increasing the plausibility of DIR has to accommodate such complex physiological motions. However, extending the spatial range of the regularization of the deformations to become less local is usually computationally prohibitive.

To overcome these limitations, this paper proposes an alternative, graph-based framework within which such non-local motion constraints, by using a range of spatial scales, can be captured naturally. Previous work in applying graph-based methods to DIR [7,8] has been primarily motivated by the use of efficient discrete optimization for minimizing the data term cost, with less focus on the regularization aspects, which are generally reduced to a fixed scale in a local regularization term. In contrast, here we show how graphical methods enable complex regularization constraints to be incorporated easily and naturally, thus improving on the plausibility of DIR algorithms in general. To introduce our approach in a familiar setting, we show how it can be applied to the classic Thirion's Demons registration [2,3], as an exemplar. Furthermore, the proposed method can easily perform non-local regularization using a minimum spanning tree (MST) derived from a graph representing the desired properties.

This work presents the use of a novel graph-based regularization model for continuous image registration based on Demons as an exemplar [2,3]. The motivation for the use of graphs stems from their ability to represent complex connected structures in a perceptually meaningful way. Such structures and connections between them can be represented for example by a MST, which has been shown to replicate well the underlying tissue properties and structure of anatomical connectivity [8]. In contrast to recently proposed anisotropic filter [4], bilateral filter [9], and guided image filter [6] models, the proposed new regularization model implicitly extends local filter kernels to their non-local counterparts by simultaneous consideration of spatial and intensity proximity together with the connectivity of voxel-based nodes. The new MST-based model replaces the Gaussian smoothing originally incorporated in Thirion's Demons [2,3] via employing an efficient MST non-local cost aggregation algorithm [10] to perform regularization on the estimated displacement field. The results achieved by our method on benchmark lung CT data [11] are compared against the best performing Demons [4–6], and a discrete MST optimization framework (deeds) [8].

2   Methods

2.1   Deformable Image Registration

Deformable image registration (DIR) is generally formulated as the minimization problem of a global energy ξ:

$$\hat{\boldsymbol{u}} = \arg \min_{\boldsymbol{u}} \left(\xi(\boldsymbol{u}) = Sim\left(R, S, \boldsymbol{u}\right) + \alpha Reg\left(\boldsymbol{u}\right) \right) \tag{1}$$

where the (optimal) displacement field $\hat{u}$ describes the geometrical transformation between two images: the reference image R and the source image S. Here, Sim measures similarity between S and R, while the regularization term Reg encourages the plausibility of the estimated displacement field u, and $\alpha \geq 0$ balances the contribution between those two terms. As an example of many, the Demons framework [2] solves the energy given in Eq. (1) in an iterative manner by alternating between minimizing similarity Sim, and regularization Reg, which performs Gaussian smoothing on the estimated displacement field. For a number of medical applications, the Demons algorithm, including the Gaussian regularization, provides very reasonable transformations [3]. However, it has been found less suitable in situations with more complex deformations. Therefore, the anisotropic [4], bilateral-like [5], and guided filter [6] regularization models have been proposed. Although the use of such regularizers considerably improves performance, it remains the case that such approaches perform regularization considering only the predefined local neighborhood around the point of interest, despite the fact that some organs can also deform in a non-local manner. In such cases, neither global nor local regularization models are sufficiently versatile to handle the complexity of the organ motion. To the best of our knowledge, incorporating connections between different anatomical structures has not been considered so far for registration regularization except for the case of registering each presegmented region separately [12].

In the next section, we show how graph-based regularization provides a mathematical framework within which local, semi-local, and global constraints can be accommodated in a natural manner. To introduce the method, we use as an exemplar the widely known and used Demons algorithm [2,3]. However, it is important to note that the method would also apply to other DIR algorithm that can be formulated as an energy minimization as above.

2.2 Graph-Based Regularization for the Demons Algorithm

The overall algorithmic approach may be summarized as follows:

1. calculate the Demons force term (classic step [2,3])
2. create a graph-based representation for the regularization model
3. find a minimum spanning tree (MST) for this graph
4. perform regularization based on MST via fast tree-cost-aggregation

Step 1 is the classic step, and is described in [2,3]. Steps 2, 3, and 4 form the new contributions of this work and will be described in detail in the following sections.

Step 2: Graph-Based Representation for Regularization. In analogy to [8], we represent the image as a graph, to accommodate the complexity of anatomical structures and connections between them. For this purpose, a graph $G = (V, E)$ is defined comprising a set of nodes V and a set of edges E. In this paper, for clarity of exposition, the nodes $p, q \in V$ are assumed to correspond to voxels of the image volume I_G, and the edges $e \in E$ connect all nearest neighbor nodes (simple 6-connected graph for a 3D volume) with the edge weight given as the absolute difference between the intensity of the node p and the respective voxel in node q. However, it has to be understood that the method applies far more generally. An exemplar graph generated for a coronal slice of a lung CT is illustrated in Fig. 1. Although only the nearest neighbor connections are considered, it will be shown later in this work that such connections can extend regularization to a non-local scale in contrast to conventional regularization methods.

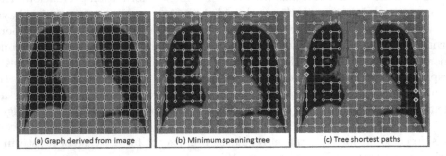

Fig. 1. Visualization of (a) graph derived from image, (b) minimum spanning tree extracted from graph (a), and (c) shortest paths between two nodes in the same (red) and different (magenta) anatomical structures. (Color figure online)

Step 3: Finding a Minimum Spanning Tree. To find a minimum spanning tree (MST) for the weighted graph G constructed in the previous section, a greedy Prim-Jarnik (P-J) algorithm is used. The P-J algorithm successively removes any unwanted edges with underlying high intensity differences from the graph, while leaving the edges connecting all nodes in the graph in the form of a tree. In practice, edges with large weights often mark edges crossing different organs, and removing them is thus advantageous in order to avoid regularization across organ boundaries. An exemplar of MST is shown in Fig. 1(b), generated from the graph presented in Fig. 1(a) of a 2D coronal slice of a lung CT. Fig. 1(c) shows the shortest path between different nodes of the graph. As can be seen, the nodes inside the same structure (red) have a short tree distance, whereas nodes within two different structures have a long tree distance despite being spatially close (magenta). Effectively, tree distance is intrinsically more relevant to regularization and deformable registration than is a spatial distance metric such as Euclidean or city block. The tree distance $\delta(p, q)$ in the constructed MST is the sum of lengths of the edges between node p and q, where the length of an edge is the Euclidean distance between the two connected nodes (for simplicity the distance between neighbor nodes is defined to be 1).

Step 4: Regularization Based on MST via Fast Tree-Cost-Aggregation.
The final step of incorporating the new graph-based regularization model to the
exemplar Demons framework combines a fast guided image filtering procedure
[13] with an efficient non-local cost aggregation algorithm for MST [10]. First, a
minimum spanning tree average operator μ^t (where ^{t} refers to tree) of variable
X is defined as follows:

$$\mu_p^t[X] = \frac{\sum_{q \in V} w(p,q) X(q)}{\sum_{q \in V} w(p,q)} \tag{2}$$

where $w(p,q) = \exp\left(-\frac{\delta(p,q)}{\sigma}\right)$ denotes a spatial tree similarity (or weight), and
σ is a weighting parameter. Direct implementation of the MST average operator
μ^t (Eq. (2)) is impractical due to the computational cost required to compute the
distances between all nodes in the graph. For this reason, Yang [10] proposed
an efficient MST cost aggregation algorithm, which requires only two passes
through the MST (two additions and three multiplications in total) in order to
calculate $\sum_{q \in V} w(p,q) X(q)$. In this paper, we employ this MST cost-aggregation
algorithm to perform regularization of the estimated displacement field $\boldsymbol{u}$. In this
way, the MST average operator μ^t replaces the standard mean operation in the
guided image filter. The guided filter is a local linear model between the guidance
image I_G and the filter output $\boldsymbol{u}_{out}$ as in our case we consider displacement field
$\boldsymbol{u}_{out}$ to be the output, and $\boldsymbol{u}_{in}$ to be the input (we refer a reader to [13] for the
detailed derivation of A and B given in Eq. 4). The guided filter is defined as
follows [13]:

$$\boldsymbol{u}_{out}(p) - \mu_p^t[A] I_G(p) + \mu_p^t[B] \tag{3}$$

where:

$$A(p) = \frac{\mu_p^t[I_G \boldsymbol{u}_{in}] - \mu_p^t[I_G] \mu_p^t[\boldsymbol{u}_{in}]}{\sigma_p^t[I_G] + \epsilon}, B(p) = \mu_p^t[\boldsymbol{u}_{in}] - A(p)\mu_p^t[I_G] \tag{4}$$

$\sigma_p^t[I_G] = \mu_p^t[I_G^2] - (\mu_p^t[I_G])^2$ is a minimum spanning tree variance, and $\epsilon > 0$
is a guided filter parameter. Considering the guidance image I_G, the output
displacement field $\boldsymbol{u}_{out}$ can be filtered with respect to the registered image (*self-
guidance*), or sparse image representation based on supervoxel clustering of the
entire thoracic cage [6]. Note that unlike anisotropic [4], guided [6] or bilateral
[5] filters, our graph-based method evaluates contributions from **all nodes** in
the graph (volume) to the estimated displacement field during the MST cost
aggregation. This substantially improves the regularization model as non-local
MST contributions can be captured simply and naturally for the whole structure
of interest, whereas the local regularization methods are limited to the (explicit)
predefined region of interest only. Although, in theory, we could extend the
predefined local patch in [4–6] to cover the full volume (however in practice
this would be computationally expensive), here the MST provides an implicit
support region without decreasing the overall efficiency.

To visualize the key differences between the local regularization models and
the proposed non-local MST method, exemplar kernels for the bilateral model
[5], and the proposed non-local MST model are shown in Fig. 2.

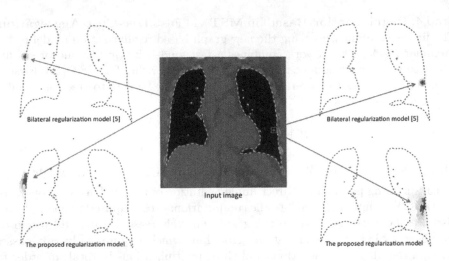

Fig. 2. Comparison between two different kernels based on input image for the local model [5], and the proposed non-local regularization model for two distinctive areas selected inside (red cross) and outside the thoracic cage (magenta cross). The implicit support region for the proposed method can efficiently present the structure of an image contrary to the predefined local region support of [5]. (Color figure online)

3   Evaluation and Results

Data. The presented method is evaluated using a publicly available 4D CT data set [11]. The *Dir-Lab* data set consists of 10 consecutive respiratory cycle phase volumes with spatial resolution varying between $0.97{\times}0.97{\times}2.5$ and $1.16{\times}1.16{\times}2.5\,\mathrm{mm}^3$. To quantify the registration accuracy, the Target Registration Error (TRE) was calculated for the well-distributed set of landmarks, which are provided with this data set (300 landmarks per case for inhale and exhale volumes). In all cases, the end-inhale image was selected as the target image and the end-exhale image as the moving image.

Implementation. For quantitative evaluation of the proposed regularization model, the Demons approach with an update composition scheme and Thirion's symmetric force was implemented (see [3] for details). For simplicity, the proposed method used the Sum of Squared Differences as a similarity measure (also used in [3–6]). The following parameters were used for the proposed registration method: $\sigma = 2.5$ (Eq. (2)), and $\epsilon = 0.1$ (Eq. (4)).

Quantitative Results and Comparison. Table 1 shows the TRE based on 300 well-populated, manually annotated landmarks for all ten cases included in the Dir-Lab data set [11]. The initial TRE is $8.46 \pm 5.5\,\mathrm{mm}$ and the transformations estimated by the proposed method reduce the TRE to $1.44 \pm 1.4\,\mathrm{mm}$, achieving the best result in our comparison. The task of registering these lung CT

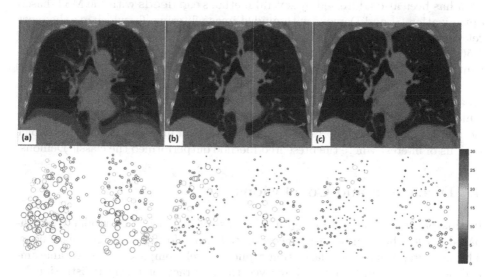

Fig. 3. Visualization of the image intensity differences (top) and 2D projection of the Target Registration Error (bottom) before registration (a), and after performing (b) classic Demons [3], and (c) the presented method for the most challenging case 8 from Dir-Lab. Color overlay is given for the coronal view of inhale (green) and exhale (magenta) volumes. TRE is projected on the coronal plane and denoted by the size and color of circles. A clear improvement after registration using the presented method is visible. (Color figure online)

Table 1. Results achieved by the proposed method (MST) and four other most relevant methods for 3D registration of CT lung from Dir-Lab data set. The proposed method shows the lowest average Target Registration Error (TRE) among all methods.

	Before	dem [3]	bil [5]	deeds [8]	gui [6]	ani [4]	MST
$c1$	3.89 ± 2.9	1.08 ± 0.6	1.05 ± 0.5	0.98 ± 0.5	1.08 ± 0.5	1.06 ± 0.6	$\mathbf{0.83 \pm 0.9}$
$c2$	4.34 ± 3.9	1.11 ± 0.6	1.08 ± 0.6	0.95 ± 0.5	1.06 ± 0.5	1.45 ± 1.0	$\mathbf{0.87 \pm 0.9}$
$c3$	6.94 ± 4.1	1.51 ± 0.9	1.46 ± 0.9	1.18 ± 0.7	1.16 ± 0.6	1.88 ± 1.4	$\mathbf{1.10 \pm 1.1}$
$c4$	9.83 ± 4.9	2.21 ± 1.8	2.05 ± 1.5	$\mathbf{1.60 \pm 1.4}$	2.11 ± 2.2	2.04 ± 1.4	1.96 ± 2.0
$c5$	7.48 ± 5.5	2.21 ± 1.9	2.02 ± 1.7	1.72 ± 1.5	1.40 ± 1.2	2.73 ± 2.1	$\mathbf{1.36 \pm 1.4}$
$c6$	10.9 ± 7.0	2.98 ± 2.6	2.48 ± 1.8	$\mathbf{1.72 \pm 1.1}$	2.21 ± 2.6	2.72 ± 2.0	1.77 ± 1.6
$c7$	11.0 ± 7.4	3.58 ± 3.5	2.78 ± 2.3	1.79 ± 1.4	1.48 ± 1.1	4.59 ± 3.4	$\mathbf{1.58 \pm 1.3}$
$c8$	15.0 ± 9.0	7.62 ± 8.1	3.96 ± 3.8	2.24 ± 2.6	2.29 ± 2.7	6.22 ± 5.7	$\mathbf{2.08 \pm 2.4}$
$c9$	7.92 ± 4.0	2.29 ± 1.7	1.89 ± 1.2	1.45 ± 0.8	$\mathbf{1.37 \pm 0.8}$	2.32 ± 1.4	1.50 ± 1.2
$c10$	7.30 ± 6.4	2.54 ± 3.1	2.35 ± 2.5	1.59 ± 1.6	1.46 ± 1.3	2.82 ± 2.5	$\mathbf{1.40 \pm 1.4}$
$T\bar{R}E$	8.46 ± 5.5	2.71 ± 1.9	2.11 ± 0.9	1.52 ± 1.4	1.56 ± 1.4	2.78 ± 2.9	$\mathbf{1.44 \pm 1.4}$

data has been also addressed by several methods e.g. **deeds** with the MST-based optimization [8] and Demons with guided image filtering [6], which are the most relevant methods for comparison, achieving a higher TRE of 1.52 ± 1.4 mm, and 1.56 ± 1.4 mm, respectively. Moreover, the proposed method achieved a significantly lower TRE ($p < 0.01$) when compared to the classic Demons registration, which only achieved a TRE of 2.71 ± 1.9 mm. Finally, Demons using anisotropic [4] and bilateral filtering [5] obtained a TRE of 2.79 ± 2.9 mm and 2.11 ± 0.9 mm, which is also inferior to the TRE obtained by the presented method. Visualization of the results for the presented method is shown in Fig. 3. Red arrows depict regions of interest where the presented method outperformed the classic Demons.

4   Discussion and Conclusions

In this paper, we have presented a new class of regularization model, a graph-based model, that can be easily incorporated into deformable image registration. The new graph-based regularization replicates well complex connected anatomical structures, and therefore improves the accuracy of image registration by implicitly estimating plausible transformations. Furthermore, the use of the efficient minimum spanning tree cost aggregation algorithm extends the predefined local support for regularization to its non-local counterpart. The quantitative evaluation on a publicly available lung CT data set confirmed superiority of the presented registration framework compared to the competing methods in the literature. Future work will include incorporation of prior knowledge combining both structural and functional imaging data coming from PET/CT or PET/MRI system to construct more complex graphs representing underlying characteristics of different organs.

Acknowledgments. We would like to acknowledge funding from the CRUK/EPSRC Cancer Imaging Centre in Oxford.

References

1. Sotiras, A., Davatzikos, C., Paragios, N.: Deformable medical image registration: a survey. IEEE Trans. Med. Imaging **32**(7), 1153–1190 (2013)
2. Thirion, J.P.: Image matching as a difusion process: an analogy with maxwell's demons. Med. Image Anal. **2**(3), 243–260 (1998)
3. Vercauteren, T., Pennec, X., Perchant, A., Ayache, N.: Difeomorphic demons: efficient non-parametric image registration. NeuroImage **45**, S61–S72 (2009)
4. Pace, D.F., Aylward, S., Niethammer, M.: A locally adaptive regularization based on anisotropic difusion for deformable image registration of sliding organs. IEEE Trans. Med. Imag. **32**(11), 2114–2126 (2013)
5. Papież, B.W., Heinrich, M.P., Fehrenbach, J., Risser, L., Schnabel, J.: An implicit sliding-motion preserving regularisation via bilateral filtering for deformable image registration. Med. Image Anal. **18**(8), 1299–1311 (2014)

6. Papież, B.W., Franklin, J., Heinrich, M.P., Gleeson, F.V., Schnabel, J.A.: Liver motion estimation via locally adaptive over-segmentation regularization. In: Navab, N., Hornegger, J., Wells, W.M., Frangi, A.F. (eds.) MICCAI 2015. LNCS, vol. 9351, pp. 427–434. Springer, Cham (2015). doi:10.1007/978-3-319-24574-4_51
7. Glocker, B., Sotiras, A., Komodakis, N., Paragios, N.: Deformable medical image registration: setting the state of the art with discrete methods. Annu. Rev. Biomed. Eng. **13**, 219–244 (2011)
8. Heinrich, M.P., Jenkinson, M., Brady, M., Schnabel, J.: MRF-based deformable registration and ventilation estimation of lung CT. IEEE Trans. Med. Imag. **32**(7), 1239–1248 (2013)
9. Papież, B.W., Heinrich, M.P., Risser, L., Schnabel, J.A.: Complex lung motion estimation via adaptive bilateral filtering of the deformation field. In: Mori, K., Sakuma, I., Sato, Y., Barillot, C., Navab, N. (eds.) MICCAI 2013. LNCS, vol. 8151, pp. 25–32. Springer, Heidelberg (2013). doi:10.1007/978-3-642-40760-4_4
10. Yang, Q.: Stereo matching using tree filtering. IEEE Trans. Pattern Anal. Mach. Intell. **37**(4), 834–846 (2015)
11. Castillo, R., Castillo, E., Guerra, R., Johnson, V.E., McPhail, T., Garg, A.K., Guerrero, T.: A framework for evaluation of deformable image registration spatial accuracy using large landmark point sets. Phys. Med. Biol. **54**, 1849–1870 (2009)
12. Wu, Z., Rietzel, E., Boldea, V., Sarrut, D., Sharp, G.: Evaluation of deformable registration of patient lung 4DCT with subanatomical region segmentations. Med. Phys. **35**(2), 775–781 (2008)
13. Dai, L., Yuan, M., Zhang, F., Zhang, X.: Fully connected guided image filtering. IEEE International Conference on Computer Vision, pp. 352–360 (2015)

Unsupervised Framework for Consistent Longitudinal MS Lesion Segmentation

Saurabh Jain[1]([⊠]), Annemie Ribbens[1], Diana M. Sima[1], Sabine Van Huffel[2], Frederik Maes[2], and Dirk Smeets[1]

[1] Icometrix, R&D, Leuven, Belgium
saurabh.jain@icometrix.com
[2] Department of Electrical Engineering-ESAT,
KU Leuven, Leuven, Belgium

Abstract. Quantification of white matter lesion changes on brain magnetic resonance (MR) images is of major importance for the follow-up of patients with Multiple Sclerosis (MS). Many automated segmentation methods have been proposed. However, most of them focus on a single time point MR scan session and hence lack consistency when evaluating lesion changes over time. In this paper, we present MSmetrix-long, an unsupervised method that incorporates temporal consistency by jointly segmenting MS lesions of two subsequent scan sessions. The method is formulated as a Maximum A Posteriori model on the FLAIR image intensities of both time points and the difference image intensities, and optimised using an expectation maximisation algorithm. Validation is performed on two different data sets in terms of consistency and sensitivity to MS lesion changes. It is shown that MSmetrix-long outperforms MSmetrix-cross for the quantification of MS lesion evolution over time.

Keywords: Longitudinal analysis · Lesion segmentation · Expectation - maximisation · Magnetic resonance imaging

1 Introduction

Accurate and reliable quantification of lesion evolution over time in patients suffering from Multiple Sclerosis (MS) is valuable for monitoring the disease activity in patient follow-up [1]. Although expert manual delineation of lesions is considered as gold standard, it is time consuming and often suffers from intra- and inter-observer variability. To alleviate these problems, automated methods for MS lesion segmentation have been proposed in literature [2–5, 7]. Many methods focus on segmentation of the lesions at a specific time point using images from a single scan session [2]. Although these methods might produce accurate lesion segmentations, they are often not suited for detecting lesion changes due to their lack of temporal consistency.

Several different longitudinal methods have also been proposed [3–7]. A first group of such methods detects longitudinal changes by time series analysis,

© Springer International Publishing AG 2017
H. Müller et al. (Eds.): MCV/BAMBI 2016, LNCS 10081, pp. 208–219, 2017.
DOI: 10.1007/978-3-319-61188-4_19

assuming long-time follow-up of the same patient (e.g. [3]). A second group of methods is also suited for follow-up between only two subsequent time points [4–7]. In [4] a registration-based approach is proposed to evaluate lesion changes between subsequent scans. However, the method requires a locally very accurate nonrigid registration as the registrations are evaluated in small regions, i.e. the lesions. Moreover, such registration-based approaches are not ideally suited in the presence of new or disappearing lesions. In [5], a method is proposed for change detection based on logistic regression models and subtraction images from consecutive time points. This method focuses, however, purely on the changes and does not allow identification of the total lesion load at both time points. More recently, two methods were proposed that focus on temporal evolution of MS lesions, including new and disappearing lesions, while also providing the segmentation of the individual time points [6,7]. The method proposed in [6] performs spectral clustering of a graph that represents spatial and temporal affinities. This method is mainly based on the image intensities and does not include information of the underlying anatomy within the segmentation process. The underlying anatomy contains however important information that can further improve the segmentation process, e.g. different intensities in juxta-cortical lesions, typical regions of pulsation artefacts on the FLAIR image, etc. Moreover, the method requires the determination of the size of spatial and temporal neighbourhoods, which may have an important impact on its performance. The method proposed in [7] focuses on the detection of new lesions using a two-step classification process, (1) a Bayesian classifier for the tissue classification and (2) final identification of new lesions based on a random-forest classification. However, this method is supervised as it requires prior learning of different aspects, such as an intensity likelihood and transition model of the lesions, from a training data set. Such a training data set needs to be representative for the population under study for these different aspects.

In this paper, we present a fully automated, unsupervised method for MS lesion evolution between two time points. The method uses both intensity information and information of the underlying anatomy. It allows the detection and segmentation of new, enlarging, disappearing, shrinking and static lesions. The method builds on an untrained cross-sectional (i.e. single time point) method, called MSmetrix-cross, that was indicated as the best untrained method in the ISBI challenge [2] and was comparable to top supervised methods.

2   Method

Our method jointly segments MS lesions of two time points based on 3D T1-weighted and 3D FLAIR images acquired at each time point. A difference image is generated to detect similar regions and changes, and as such to introduce temporal consistency or to allow flexibility between the segmentations of both time points. Prior knowledge on the tissue classes and MS lesions will be included by performing first a cross-sectional segmentation method per time point, called MSmetrix-cross. In the next sections, we describe the pipeline of MSmetrix-long, i.e. (1) a preprocessing step, including (a) generation of tissue prior probabilities based on MSmetrix-cross, and (b) the difference image, (2) joint segmentation formulated by a Maximum a Posteriori (MAP) problem and (3) a pruning step.

All steps will be performed in two spaces, i.e. first for the image of time point 1 which is used as reference space and subsequently for the image of time point 2. Our method iterates three times between both spaces taking each time the lesion segmentation from the previous iteration as input for the new iteration. These iterations are performed to avoid bias towards one of both time points. An overview of the method is shown in Fig. 1.

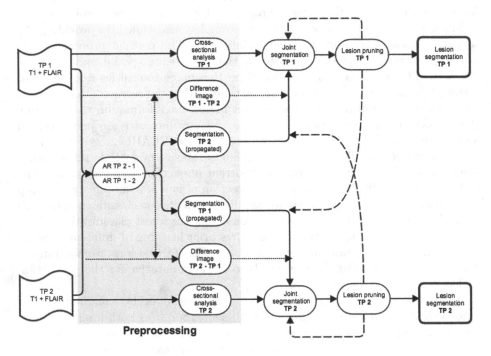

Fig. 1. Schematic representation of the MSmetrix-long pipeline. Notations: TP is time point, AR is affine registration.

2.1   Preprocessing

Cross-sectional analysis: Image segmentation is performed independently for each time point using a cross-sectional segmentation pipeline [8]. First, the FLAIR image is resampled towards the space of the T1-weighted image using a rigid registration. The cross-sectional method then segments the T1-weighted image into the normal brain tissue classes, i.e. grey matter (GM), white matter (WM) and cerebro-spinal fluid (CSF) using an Expectation Maximisation (EM) algorithm. Subsequently, it segments the WM lesions in the FLAIR image as outliers to the intensities of the normal brain tissue classes obtained from the

T1-weighted image segmentation. A pruning step [8] is performed to distinguish FLAIR WM lesions from other outliers. Finally, a lesion filling of the T1-weighted image is performed. These steps are iteratively performed until convergence. As such, probabilistic segmentations for GM, WM, CSF and the FLAIR WM lesions are obtained. In addition, the method produces bias field corrected T1-weighted and FLAIR images.

Difference image: A difference image of the bias field corrected FLAIR images is created by image co-registration and intensity normalisation. Co-registration between the images of both time points is performed, as described in [9], using a symmetric affine registration with the scaling step based on the extracted skull. The matched bias corrected FLAIR images are then corrected for a differential bias field as described in [10] and thereafter, intensity normalised using a cumulative histogram matching technique [11]. A difference image is now created in the reference space.

Propagation: The segmentations obtained from the cross-sectional analysis are resampled towards the reference space using the same affine registration as used to create the difference image.

2.2   Joint Lesion Segmentation

We now define a model that aims at joint tissue class label segmentation based on the co-registered FLAIR images of both time points and the difference image.

Notations: Denote $Y^{(1)} = \{y_j^{(1)} | j \in \{1, \ldots, N_J\}\}$, $Y^{(2)} = \{y_j^{(2)} | j \in \{1, \ldots, N_J\}\}$ and $Y^{(D)} = \{y_j^{(D)} | j \in \{1, \ldots, N_J\}\}$ the sets of image intensities of resp. the FLAIR image of time point 1, the FLAIR image of time point 2 and the difference image, with $y_j^{(1)}$, $y_j^{(2)}$ and $y_j^{(D)}$ the image intensities corresponding to voxel j in the corresponding image and N_J the voxel size (assumed to be the same in every image after co-registration). We assume that the total number of tissue classes in both images is equal and denoted by N_K. The tissue class labels for resp. image 1 and 2 can be denoted by $L^{(1)} = \{l_{j,k^{(1)}}^{(1)}\}$ and $L^{(2)} = \{l_{j,k^{(2)}}^{(2)}\}$ with $k^{(1)}$ and $k^{(2)} \in \{1, \ldots, N_K\}$ the tissue class indices. In this paper, the tissue classes will be GM, WM, CSF and lesions.

Model assumptions: The intensities of image 1 can be modelled as a Gaussian mixture model over the tissue classes with parameter set $\theta^{(1)}$ representing the set of means $(\mu_{k^{(1)}}^{(1)})$ and variances $(\sigma_{k^{(1)}}^{2(1)})$ of all Gaussians:

$$P(Y^{(1)} | L^{(1)}, \theta^{(1)}) = \prod_{j,k^{(1)}} \mathcal{N}\left(y_j^{(1)} | \mu_{k^{(1)}}^{(1)}, \sigma_{k^{(1)}}^{2(1)}\right)^{l_{j,k^{(1)}}^{(1)}} \tag{1}$$

Analogously, we can model the intensities of the image 2 as:

$$P(Y^{(2)} | L^{(2)}, \theta^{(2)}) = \prod_{j,k^{(2)}} \mathcal{N}\left(y_j^{(2)} | \mu_{k^{(2)}}^{(2)}, \sigma_{k^{(2)}}^{2(2)}\right)^{l_{j,k^{(2)}}^{(2)}} \tag{2}$$

We make the underlying assumption that the "difference image" might be independently generated as an image that captures anatomical changes including new lesions or atrophy. The image created by subtracting image 1 from image 2 or vice-versa (after intensity normalisation) is one such instance of the difference image. The intensity model of image 1 and image 2 can therefore be improved by including a transition model defined on the difference image. As our major interest is in the WM lesion segmentation, we only model the transitions between WM and lesions and hence assume a uniform distribution for transitions between all other tissue classes. For the transitions between WM and lesions, we use a Gaussian mixture model on the intensities with three different classes, *i.e.* static, lesion growth and lesion shrinkage. The static transition class is defined as a set of voxels in the difference image that are either labeled as WM in both images or as lesions in both images. The lesion growth class is defined as the transition between the WM label in image 1 and the lesion label in image 2. The lesion shrinkage class is defined as the transition between the lesion label in image 1 and the WM label in image 2. Hence, our transition model $P(Y^{(D)}|L^{(1)}, L^{(2)}, \zeta)$ can be defined as:

$$P(Y^{(D)}|L^{(1)}, L^{(2)}, \zeta) = \begin{cases} \propto 1 & \text{, with } k^{(1)} \text{ and } k^{(2)} \in \{\text{GM, CSF}\} \\ \prod_{j,k^{(1)},k^{(2)}} \mathcal{N}\left(y_j^{(D)}|\mu_{k^{(1)},k^{(2)}}^{(D)}, \sigma_{k^{(1)},k^{(2)}}^{2(D)}\right)^{l_{j,k^{(1)}}^{(1)} \cdot l_{j,k^{(2)}}^{(2)}} & \text{, with } k^{(1)} \text{ and } k^{(2)} \in \{\text{WM, lesion}\} \end{cases}$$

(3)

where $\zeta = \{\theta_{static}, \theta_{growth}, \theta_{shrinkage}\}$ the set of Gaussian mixture parameters of the three transition classes with

$$\theta_{static} = \{\mu_{k^{(1)},k^{(2)}}^{(D)}, \sigma_{k^{(1)},k^{(2)}}^{2(D)}\}, \qquad \text{if} \begin{cases} k^{(1)} = k^{(2)} = \text{WM or} \\ k^{(1)} = k^{(2)} = \text{lesion} \end{cases}$$

$$\theta_{growth} = \{\mu_{k^{(1)},k^{(2)}}^{(D)}, \sigma_{k^{(1)},k^{(2)}}^{2(D)}\}, \qquad \text{if } k^{(1)} = \text{WM}, k^{(2)} = \text{lesion}$$

$$\theta_{shrinkage} = \{\mu_{k^{(1)},k^{(2)}}^{(D)}, \sigma_{k^{(1)},k^{(2)}}^{2(D)}\}, \quad \text{if } k^{(1)} = \text{lesion}, k^{(2)} = \text{WM}$$

Finally, we assume that we have no prior knowledge on the relationship on the tissue class labels between both images. Therefore, we define the prior probabilities independently for each image. Often these prior probabilities are given by a probabilistic atlas. However, our cross-sectional model provided us with more specific knowledge and hence, we use the probabilistic cross-sectional tissue class segmentations. The prior probabilities on tissue class labels for image 1 is denoted by $P(L^{(1)})$ and for the image 2 is denoted by $P(L^{(2)})$, are defined as:

$$P(L^{(1)}) = \prod_{j,k^{(1)}} \left(\alpha_{j,k^{(1)}}^{(1)}\right)^{l_{j,k^{(1)}}^{(1)}} \quad , \quad P(L^{(2)}) = \prod_{j,k^{(2)}} \left(\alpha_{j,k^{(2)}}^{(2)}\right)^{l_{j,k^{(2)}}^{(2)}} \qquad (4)$$

Maximum A Posteriori (MAP) problem: We want to optimise our model $P(\gamma|Y^{(1)}, Y^{(2)}, Y^{(D)})$ with parameters $\gamma = \{\theta_1, \theta_2, \zeta\}$ to fit the observed image intensities $Y^{(1)}$, $Y^{(2)}$ and $Y^{(D)}$. Hence, we aim to optimise the following MAP:

$$\gamma_{\text{MAP}} = \underset{\gamma}{argmax} \ \ln P(\gamma|Y^{(1)}, Y^{(2)}, Y^{(D)}) = \underset{\gamma}{argmax} \ \ln \ P(Y^{(1)}, Y^{(2)}, Y^{(D)}, \gamma)$$

$$(5)$$

$$= \underset{\gamma}{argmax} \ \ln \sum_{L^{(1)}, L^{(2)}} P(Y^{(1)}, Y^{(2)}, Y^{(D)}, L^{(1)}, L^{(2)}, \gamma) \qquad (6)$$

$$\geq \underset{\gamma}{argmax} \sum_{L^{(1)}, L^{(2)}} P(L^{(1)}, L^{(2)}|Y^{(1)}, Y^{(2)}, Y^{(D)}, \overline{\gamma}) \ \ln \ \frac{P(Y^{(1)}, Y^{(2)}, Y^{(D)}, L^{(1)}, L^{(2)}, \gamma)}{P(L^{(1)}, L^{(2)}|Y^{(1)}, Y^{(2)}, Y^{(D)}, \overline{\gamma})}$$

$$(7)$$

where

$$P(Y^{(1)}, Y^{(2)}, Y^{(D)}, L^{(1)}, L^{(2)}, \gamma) = P(Y^{(1)}|L^{(1)}, \theta^{(1)}). \ P(Y^{(2)}|L^{(2)}, \theta^{(2)})$$
$$. \ P(Y^{(D)}|L^{(1)}, L^{(2)}, \zeta). \ P(L^{(1)})$$
$$. \ P(L^{(2)}) \qquad (8)$$

and Eq. (6) is introduced as knowledge of tissue class labels (hidden variables) contributes to the estimation of the model parameters. To optimise this model with hidden variables, a lower bound (Eq. (7)) is derived using Jensen's inequality. The Q-function can now be written as:

$$Q(\gamma|\overline{\gamma}) = \ E_{L^{(1)}, L^{(2)}|Y^{(1)}, Y^{(2)}, Y^{(D)}, \overline{\gamma}} \ [\ \ln \ P(Y^{(1)}, Y^{(2)}, Y^{(D)}, L^{(1)}, L^{(2)}, \gamma)] \quad (9)$$

with the joint posterior distribution $P(L^{(1)}, L^{(2)}|Y^{(1)}, Y^{(2)}, Y^{(D)}, \overline{\gamma})$, which can be formulated in every voxel j for tissue class $k^{(1)}$ and $k^{(2)}$ as:

$$p_{j, k^{(1)}, k^{(2)}} = \frac{p(y_j^{(1)}, y_j^{(2)}, y_j^{(D)}, l_{j, k^{(1)}}^{(1)} = 1, l_{j, k^{(2)}}^{(2)} = 1, \overline{\gamma})}{\sum\limits_{k^{(1)}, k^{(2)}} p(y_j^{(1)}, y_j^{(2)}, y_j^{(D)}, l_{j, k^{(1)}}^{(1)}, l_{j, k^{(2)}}^{(2)}, \overline{\gamma})} \qquad (10)$$

for a specific estimate $\overline{\gamma}$ of γ. Marginalisation of the joint posterior over all possible tissue classes $k^{(2)}$ provides us an estimate of the soft tissue class segmentations at time point 1, referred to as $p_{j, k^{(1)}}$. Analogously, marginalisation over all $k^{(1)}$ of the joint posterior provides us the soft tissue class segmentations at time point 2, referred to as $p_{j, k^{(2)}}$.

$$p_{j, k^{(1)}} = \sum_{k^{(2)}} p_{j, k^{(1)}, k^{(2)}} \qquad (11)$$

$$p_{j,k^{(2)}} = \sum_{k^{(1)}} p_{j,k^{(1)},k^{(2)}} \qquad (12)$$

The EM algorithm iteratively optimises the posterior distribution in the expectation step based on a parameter estimation obtained from the maximisation step. In the maximisation step, the parameters are updated by maximisation of the lower bound in Eq. (9) for the current estimate of the joint posterior. Closed form solutions for all parameters are found.

2.3   Pruning

The obtained segmentations from the EM algorithm are evaluated to check whether they fulfil the criteria for MS lesions: (1) the lesion intensities should be hyper-intense compared to the WM intensities on the bias field corrected FLAIR image, (2) the lesions are in the WM region, and (3) the lesion needs to have a minimum volume of 0.005 ml (empirically determined) to avoid spurious lesion detection. In addition, a priori defined binary mask that consists of the cerebral cortex and WM in-between the ventricles is warped to the subject space to remove lesion candidates from these regions as they are likely to result in a false lesion segmentation.

3   Experiments and Results

The longitudinal pipeline (MSmetrix-long) is compared to the cross-sectional pipeline (MSmetrix-cross) in terms of consistency and sensitivity in lesion evolution. In-house data sets are used as the publicly available ISBI challenge is not ideally suited for evaluating consistency (as no test-retest data available) or sensitivity (as almost no new lesions present in the follow-up data). Two tailed paired Wilcoxon signed-rank test is performed to detect significant differences between the results of both methods.

3.1   Consistency Experiment

The consistency of the lesion segmentation is validated on test-rest data of 10 MS patients. Each patient was scanned two times, with re-positioning, on each of three different 3T scanners (i.e. Philips, Siemens and GE). Each scan session contained a 3D FLAIR and a 3D T1-weighted image with voxel resolution close to $1\,mm^3$. No expert segmentations are available. The consistency of both MSmetrix-cross and MSmetrix-long is evaluated by the Dice overlap of the lesion segmentations of both times points. Moreover, we calculate the estimated number of new lesions and the absolute total lesion volume difference from the first towards the second scan, which are both expected to be zero.

All quantitative results are visualised in Table 1. MSmetrix-long shows a significant improved Dice overlap as well as a better estimate of the number of new lesions (p-values < 0.01) compared to MSmetrix-cross. Also, the absolute volume difference between the time points is improved in the longitudinal method, although this is not significant (p-value > 0.05). Figure 2(a) shows an example of improved temporal consistency of the lesion segmentation.

Table 1. The Dice overlap, the number (nr.) of new lesions and the absolute volume difference (abs. vol. diff.) between both time points for MSmetrix-cross and MSmetrix-long. All metrics are reported as median (first quartile − third quartile).

Method	Dice	Nr. new lesions	Abs. vol. diff. (ml)
MSmetrix-cross	0.69 (0.56 − 0.73)*	3.5 (1 − 5)*	0.30 (0.17 − 0.54)
MSmetrix-long	0.89 (0.85 − 0.91)	0 (0 − 1)	0.13 (0.04 − 0.39)

* Values significantly different from MSmetrix-long (paired Wilcoxon signed-rank test with $p < 0.01$ significance level).

3.2 Sensitivity Experiment

This experiment is based on a baseline and a one-year follow-up scan from 12 MS patients on a GE 3T scanner. Each time point contained a 3D FLAIR and 3D T1-weighted image with voxel resolution close to $1\,mm^3$. Expert MS lesion segmentations are available and the number of new lesions for the data set according to the ground truth equals 4 (2.75 − 7.25) (median (first quartile − third quartile)). These new lesions (number and location) were used to evaluate the sensitivity. Hence we calculate the lesion-wise true positive rate (LTPR) and lesion-wise false positive rate (LFPR) for new lesions with respect to the ground truth [2]. LTPR is defined as the ratio of the total number of new lesions where the ground truth and the automatic segmentation intersect to the total number of new lesions in the ground truth segmentation. LFPR is defined as the ratio of the total number of new lesions that are present only in the automatic segmentation to the total number of new lesions in the automatic segmentation.

For completeness, we also compute the Dice overlap between the overall lesion segmentation of each methods and the ground truth per time point. Table 2 summarises the results. No significant differences (p-value > 0.05) are found for LTPR and the Dice scores between both methods, although the Dice scores seem slightly better for MSmetrix-long. The LFPR is significantly improved for MSmetrix-long compared to MSmetrix-cross $(p-value < 0.01)$. Figure 2(b) shows a representative example of lesion segmentation obtained by both methods, illustrating the consistency of MSmetrix-long, while still detecting the lesion changes.

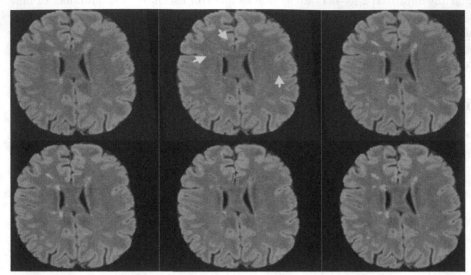

(a) Bias corrected FLAIR image with lesion segmentation from MSmetrix-cross (red) and MSmetrix-long (green).

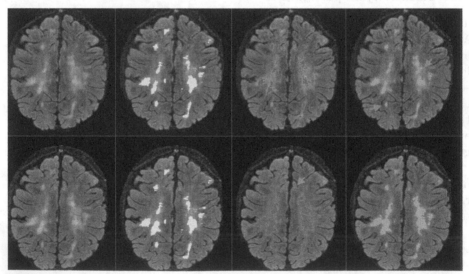

(b) Bias corrected FLAIR image with lesion segmentation from the expert (yellow), MSmetrix-cross (red) and MSmetrix-long (green).

Fig. 2. (a) Consistency and (b) sensitivity of the lesion segmentations on 2 representative examples. The first row are the time point 1 images and the second row time point 2. (Color figure online)

Table 2. The Dice overlap, LTPR and LFPR for MSmetrix-cross and MSmetrix-long with respect to expert segmentations. All metrics are reported in median (first quartile − third quartile).

Method	LTPR	LFPR	Dice TP 1	Dice TP 2
MSmetrix-cross	0.25 (0.25 − 0.38)	0.78 (0.67 − 0.93)*	0.65 (0.52 − 0.68)	0.58 (0.45 − 0.63)
MSmetrix-long	0.21 (0 − 0.38)	0.23 (0 − 0.29)	0.65 (0.54 − 0.69)	0.59 (0.47 − 0.66)

LTPR=lesion-wise true positive rate for new lesions, LFPR=lesion-wise false positive rate for new lesions, Dice=voxel-wise overlap between automated method and the ground truth lesion segmentation per time point.
* Values significantly different from MSmetrix-long (paired Wilcoxon signed-rank test with $p < 0.01$ significance level).

4   Discussion and Conclusion

We have presented MSmetrix-long: a longitudinal method for lesion joint segmentation over two time points, optimised using an EM algorithm. The proposed method is unsupervised and can segment new, enlarging, disappearing, shrinking and static lesions. The method combines both spatial and temporal relationships of lesions for accurate and consistent lesion segmentation. The spatial relationship is based on Markov Random Field and is incorporated in MSmetrix-cross. The temporal relationship is modelled in a joint lesion segmentation, which uses difference image and cross-sectional lesion segmentations of two time points. The difference image models the growth and shrinkage of lesions and thus helps in recovering those lesions that are missed in the MSmetrix-cross. In addition, if a lesion is present in both time points but has been segmented in only one of the time point, then the joint lesion segmentation facilitates the recovery of that lesion at the other time point. Moreover, brain atrophy has also minimal impact on the performance of MSmetrix-long because (1) atrophy is generally small and global in nature (2) it occurs near the CSF boundary and these transitions *i.e.* (CSF → GM and CSF → WM) are excluded in the difference image GMM model, (3) we tested global non-rigid registration *i.e.* non-rigid registration only on a coarse level, to accommodate for the atrophy and we found out that it has a minimal impact on the final lesion segmentation. Therefore, to gain computational efficiency we excluded this global non-rigid registration from MSmetrix-long pipeline.

Among the methods proposed in the literature for longitudinal lesion segmentation, our approach has some similarities to [5] and [7]. As opposed to [5], which uses four MRI sequences and their respective difference images of two consecutive time points in a logistic regression model to detect lesion changes, our method is unsupervised and works with only two clinically acquired MRI sequences. In contrast with [7], which is also based on EM framework, our method is unsupervised and can segment new, enlarging, disappearing and shrinking lesions.

One important aspect of MSmetrix-long is that its performance is dependent on the cross-sectional lesion segmentation. This suggests that if MSmetrix-cross has either consistently missed a lesion, or segmented a non-lesion at both time points, then it will be either missed or retained by MSmetrix-long, respectively. As presented in the result section, MSmetrix-long is more consistent than MSmetrix-cross and sensitive in terms of detecting lesion changes. The increase in consistency is due to the reduction in false positives using the lesion segmentation information from the other time point. A slight decrease in the sensitivity in detecting lesion changes is due to the elimination of a few lesions that are close to the cerebral cortex. Interestingly, in spite of substantial reduction in the false positive rate of new lesions, the Dice overlap for both methods remains the same (see Table 2). This can be explained by the fact that new lesions are very small and thus their impact on the overall (global) lesion segmentation Dice overlap is minimal.

We have presented MSmetrix-long: a longitudinal method for lesion joint segmentation over two time points, optimised using an EM algorithm. The proposed method is unsupervised and can segment new, enlarging, disappearing, shrinking and static lesions. The method was evaluated on two data sets in terms of temporal consistency and sensitivity to MS lesion changes. It is indicated that MSmetrix-long is more consistent than MSmetrix-cross and as sensitive in terms of detecting lesion changes. As such, MSmetrix-long allows an improved quantification of MS lesion evolution.

References

1. Blystad, I., Hakansson, I., Tisell, A., et al.: Quantitative MRI for analysis of active multiple sclerosis lesions without gadolinium-based contrast agent. Am. J. Neuroradiol. **37**, 94–100 (2016)
2. Pham, D.: The 2015 longitudinal multiple sclerosis lesion segmentation challenge, ISBI (2015). http://iacl.ece.jhu.edu/MSChallenge
3. Gerig, G., Welti, D., Guttmann, C.R.G., et al.: Exploring the discriminative power of the time domain for segmentation and characterisation of active lesions in serial MR data. Med. Image Anal. **4**, 31–42 (2000)
4. Rey, D., Subsol, G., Delingette, H., et al.: Automatic detection and segmentation of evolving processes in 3D medical images: application to multiple sclerosis. Med. Image Anal. **6**, 163–179 (2002)
5. Sweeney, E.M., Shinohara, R.T., Shea, C.D., et al.: Automatic lesion incidence estimation and detection in multiple sclerosis using multisequence longitudinal MRI. MSmetrix Am. J. Neuroradiol. **34**, 68–73 (2013)
6. Bernardis, E., Pohl, K.M., Davatzikos, C.: Extracting evolving pathologies via spectral clustering. In: Gee, J.C., Joshi, S., Pohl, K.M., Wells, W.M., Zöllei, L. (eds.) IPMI 2013. LNCS, vol. 7917, pp. 680–691. Springer, Heidelberg (2013). doi:10.1007/978-3-642-38868-2_57
7. Elliott, C., Arnold, D.L., Collins, D.L., et al.: Temporally consistent probabilistic detection of new multiple sclerosis lesions in brain MRI. IEEE Trans. Med. Imaging **32**, 1490–1503 (2013)
8. Jain, S., Sima, D.M., Ribbens, A., et al.: Automatic segmentation and volumetry of multiple sclerosis brain lesions from MR images. NeuroImage Clin. **8**, 367–375 (2015)

9. Smeets, D., Ribbens, A., Sima, D.M., et al.: Reliable measurements of brain atrophy in individual patients with multiple sclerosis. Brain Behav. 1.e00518–12.e00518 (2016). doi:10.1002/brb3.518
10. Lewis, E.B., Fox, N.C.: Correction of differential intensity inhomogeneity in longitudinal MR images. NeuroImage **23**, 75–83 (2004)
11. Castleman, K.R.: Digital Image Processing, 2nd edn. Prentice Hall, New Jersey (1995)

Employment of Innovation for Competitive Advantage [A]. London., 210

Manoj, G.P. Manager, Shop 306 ... ... refine on the copious copies of Edition ... ... fig and residing ones which ... ... works Br. in L... i... m... s. ... 1919, ... 1910, ... 10-...347, 316

Marcus, A.A. ... ... Corporate ... of Alternative Structure of Innovation it ... c...
... n... ... c... State ... ..., 53, p... ...

...gos... A.E. ... Paper...

Author Index

Printed in the United States
By Bookmasters